Register Now fo
to Youı

MW00843762

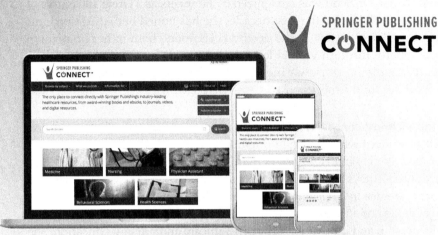

SPRINGER PUBLISHING
CƟNNECT™

Your print purchase of *Transitioning from RN to MSN*
includes online access to the contents of your book—
increasing accessibility, portability, and searchability!

Access today at:
http://connect.springerpub.com/content/book/978-0-8261-3807-1
or scan the QR code at the right with your smartphone. Log in or
register, then click "Redeem a voucher" and use the code below.

> **SB3BP455**

*Scan here for
quick access.*

Having trouble redeeming a voucher code?
Go to https://connect.springerpub.com/redeeming-voucher-code

If you are experiencing problems accessing the digital component of
this product, please contact our customer service department at cs@
springerpub.com

The online access with your print purchase is available at the publisher's discretion
and may be removed at any time without notice.

Publisher's Note: New and used products purchased from third-party sellers are not
guaranteed for quality, authenticity, or access to any included digital components.

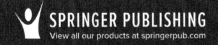

SPRINGER PUBLISHING
View all our products at springerpub.com

Brenda Scott, DNP, RN, NHDP-BC, holds bachelor's and master's degrees in nursing and completed her doctor of nursing practice in administration degree in 2015. She is also a board certified national healthcare disaster professional. Dr. Scott was recognized by her peers as a Great 100 Nurse of Arkansas in 2017. For the past decade, she has honed her education craft from the clinical setting to the doctoral classroom, both in her hometown and globally through virtual learning spaces. When she is not leading faculty teams or empowering nursing students, she devotes time to support her local American Red Cross chapter.

Mindy Thompson, DNP, RN, CNE, is a nontraditional, first-generation college student who set out in pursuit of an associate's degree in nursing to follow her calling right out of high school. She has since earned bachelor's and master's degrees in nursing and completed her doctor of nursing practice degree in 2017. With more than 20 years of collective experience at the bedside and in the classroom, Dr. Thompson has a proven track record of leadership and innovation in both healthcare and nursing education. She is a member of Sigma Theta Tau International (STTI) and has been nationally recognized with various awards and scholarships. She has served in leadership positions in both STTI chapters and her region of the Oklahoma Nurses Association. Apart from her professional and academic achievements, Dr. Thompson is committed to serving her local community. In her spare time, she volunteers with Good Samaritan Health Services to help provide healthcare services to the uninsured.

Transitioning From RN to MSN

Principles of Professional Role Development

Brenda Scott, DNP, RN, NHDP-BC

Mindy Thompson, DNP, RN, CNE

Editors

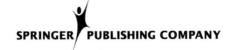

SPRINGER PUBLISHING COMPANY

Springer Publishing Company, LLC
11 West 42nd Street
New York, NY 10036
www.springerpub.com

Acquisitions Editor: Elizabeth Nieginski
Associate Managing Editor: Kris Parrish
Compositor: Graphic World

ISBN: 978-0-8261-3796-8
ebook ISBN: 978-0-8261-3807-1
Instructor's Manual: 978-0-8261-3992-4
Instructor's PowerPoints: 978-0-8261-3656-5

Instructors Materials: Qualified instructors may request supplements by emailing textbook @springerpub.com.

19 20 21 22 23 / 5 4 3 2 1

The author and the publisher of this Work have made every effort to use sources believed to be reliable to provide information that is accurate and compatible with the standards generally accepted at the time of publication. Because medical science is continually advancing, our knowledge base continues to expand. Therefore, as new information becomes available, changes in procedures become necessary. We recommend that the reader always consult current research and specific institutional policies before performing any clinical procedure. The author and publisher shall not be liable for any special, consequential, or exemplary damages resulting, in whole or in part, from the readers' use of, or reliance on, the information contained in this book. The publisher has no responsibility for the persistence or accuracy of URLs for external or third-party Internet websites referred to in this publication and does not guarantee that any content on such websites is, or will remain, accurate or appropriate.

Library of Congress Cataloging-in-Publication Data

Names: Scott, Brenda, 1983- editor. | Thompson, Mindy, 1977- editor.
Title: Transitioning from RN to MSN : principles of professional role
   development / [edited by] Brenda Scott, Mindy Thompson.
Description: New York, NY : Springer Publishing Company, LLC, [2019] |
   Includes bibliographical references and index.
Identifiers: LCCN 2018021366 (print) | LCCN 2018022483 (ebook) | ISBN
   9780826138071 | ISBN 9780826137968 (pbk.) | ISBN 9780826138071 (e-book) |
   ISBN 9780826139924 (Instructor's manual) | ISBN 9780826136565
   (Instructor's PowerPoints)
Subjects: | MESH: Nurses | Nurse's Role | Nursing, Supervisory
Classification: LCC RT82 (ebook) | LCC RT82 (print) | NLM WY 87 | DDC
   610.73—dc23
LC record available at https://lccn.loc.gov/2018021366

Contact us to receive discount rates on bulk purchases.
We can also customize our books to meet your needs.
For more information please contact: sales@springerpub.com

Printed in the United States of America.

To Jaison, with love. To Mom: thanks for sharing your passion for nursing and providing a role model for me to look up to. To Dad, who taught me the value of education and hard work.—Much love, Brenda

To Dakota and Cody: I hope my work is an inspiration for you to continue setting goals and pursuing your dreams in every area of life. What you can achieve is determined only by the extent of your dreams and your willingness to pursue them.—Love, Mom

In honor of my Mom.—Mindy

Contents

●●●●

Contributors

Lea Brandt, OTD, MA
Adjunct Associate Professor
University of Missouri School of Medicine
Center for Health Ethics
Executive Director
Missouri Health Professions Consortium
Columbia, Missouri

Amanda S. Brown, PhD, RN, CNL
Associate Director, Patient Care Services
SUNY Upstate Medical University Hospital
Syracuse, New York

Annie Donaway, PhD, RN
Course Faculty
Western Governors University
Salt Lake City, Utah

Dana Hill, PhD, RN, CPHQ
Curriculum Technology Manager
Chamberlain University
Downers Grove, Illinois

Eleanor Hunt, DNP, RN-BC
Course Faculty
Western Governors University
Salt Lake City, Utah

Gina M. Oliver, PhD, APRN, FNP-BC, CNE
Associate Teaching Professor
University of Missouri
Sinclair School of Nursing
Columbia, Missouri

Nycole Oliver, DNP, APRN, RN, FNP-C, ACNPC-AG, CEN
Nurse Practitioner
Sparks Medical Center Van Buren
Van Buren, Arkansas

Bonnie Pierce, EdD, RN, CENP
Associate Director, Patient Care Services
Eastern Oklahoma VA Health Care System
Muskogee, Oklahoma

Lori Popejoy, PhD, RN, FAAN
Associate Professor
University of Missouri
Sinclair School of Nursing
University of Missouri, Columbia

Tara Slagle, MSN, RN
Nurse Manager, Emergency Services
UPMC Pinnacle Hanover
Hanover, Pennsylvania

Foreword

As the nursing world advances the education and practice of nurses, many roles have not received as much attention and acknowledgment as others. Because of the rapid acceptance and increase in the numbers of DNP programs, some of the MSN roles and advances have not received as much attention as they probably should. This book addresses some of those gaps.

This book is an excellent introduction to nursing at the master's level. The book is composed of several sections that can be extremely helpful to nurses moving toward the next level of their careers. The first section (Foundations of Role Development in Master's-Level Nursing Education) on the history of nursing and the history of the different advanced roles in nursing is very informative. Chapter 2 (Nursing Process and Theory Selection) is succinct and appropriate for a brief introduction. There are several issues related to ethics, and although all nurses deal with ethical dilemmas, these sections are very helpful in delineating the different aspects of the subject. This book could be introduced to students at the BSN level to help them make career choices as they move forward with their careers.

For the purposes of identifying the variety of roles in which MSN students can be educated, the chapters on the different roles at the MSN level are concise yet contain the appropriate amount of detail to assist students in identifying the role to which they are best suited. There is some historic detail as well as current information about how the roles are utilized and sections on how the nurses in those roles can advance within those roles. Although there is an abundance of information about the APRN roles, there is minimal literature adequately summarizing other roles such as informatics and the nurse executive. The materials included in these sections can be helpful not only to the student in those roles but also to other MSN students.

Chapter 11 makes it clear that the MSN-prepared nurse must plan to assist in making changes. Those changes may be in the system, population health, or individual practice on the basis of evidence, but the role mandates that nurses be change managers. The other area in which the book has good applicable information is in the area of quality and ethical dilemmas. In addition, nursing leadership and the MSN role in change and team-based activities are discussed. These areas are the current focus of all MSN-prepared nurses and are extremely important to the role of nurses who plan to advance their careers. Chapter 16, on mentoring, likewise can be helpful to all nurses, both at the MSN level and at the BSN level.

Chapter 16 delineates the differences between the MSN-prepared nurse and the BSN-prepared nurse on the basis of the AACN Essentials at each level. This chapter gives examples of the differences in role expectations and responsibilities between the BSN- and MSN-prepared nurse. In addition, Chapter 13 discusses the role of interprofessional care and the need for team care that has been identified by the Institute of Medicine (IOM) as being the best way to improve patient care (IOM, 2001). Finally, the role of mentorship is discussed, both as a mentor and as a mentee. Mentorship has received much discussion nationally, but this section is a succinct discussion of how to navigate the mentor and mentee roles.

One of the most important sections of each chapter is the Critical Thinking Questions. Chapter 14 makes the vital statement that all nurses be lifelong learners, and the critical thinking questions spur the reader to move beyond the knowledge that is presented to the possibilities opened to them in the critical thinking questions. Having a potential clinical nurse leader (CNL) or nurse leader consider the differences and similarities in roles is hugely beneficial when one is planning one's career. Trying to put to use the different types of theories and apply them to one's current setting makes them seem more real.

Carol L. Savrin DNP, CPNP, PC, FNP-BC, FAANP, FNAP
Associate Professor of Nursing
Case Western Reserve University
Cleveland, Ohio

REFERENCE

Institute of Medicine. (2001). *Crossing the quality chasm: A new health system for the 21st century*. Washington, DC: National Academies Press.

Foreword

●●●●

As pratitioners of one of the single largest health professions in the country and for the past 16 years the most ethical and respected professional group (Brenan, 2017), one would expect nurses and their practice to be well understood. Unfortunately, there still exist huge gaps of knowledge and understanding about the roles and contributions nurses make in contemporary society.

At the time of writing this book, there are more than 3.5 million nurses in the United States working in countless specialties in settings ranging from hospitals to clinics to communities and homes. Nurses provide direct patient care, conduct research, teach, lead, innovate, and make policy for the advancement of the health of our nation. Despite the amazing depth and breadth of contributions made by nurses, there is a gap in the literature describing not only the history and theoretical foundations from which the profession has evolved but also the contemporary roles, in particular, for nurses prepared at the graduate level.

The differentiation of nursing from other health professionals, in particular, medicine, has often been misstated and mistaken for a second or lesser career choice. What readers will find in this book are the reasons why individuals should choose nursing first and why they can be so confident in the knowledge that they are choosing a diverse, intellectually challenging, socially relevant, and personally gratifying career. The opportunities and alternatives for nurses have never been greater. The personal and career benefits are wide ranging. This book gives every nurse or potential nurse a picture of possibility and a vision for a satisfying and sustainable career.

Dr. Jan Jones-Schenk, D.HSc, RN, NE-BC
Academic Vice President, College of Health Professions
Western Governors University
Past President, American Nurses Credentialing Center

REFERENCE

Brenan, M. (2017, December 26). Nurses keep healthy lead as most honest, ethical profession. *Gallup News.* Retrieved from https://news.gallup.com/poll/224639/nurses-keep-healthy-lead-honest-ethical-profession.aspx?g_source=Economy&g_medium=newsfeed&g_campaign=tiles

Preface

••••

Our purpose for creating this book was to address a gap in literature regarding nonadvanced practice nursing degrees. Most of the MSN role transition books on the market have a heavy focus on the advanced practice registered nurse role. Although we appreciate the need for these types of books, we saw the need to address other roles MSN-prepared nurses pursue. We focused on key roles in both direct and indirect care settings as identified by the American Association of Colleges of Nursing.

We also felt a need to take a different approach in explaining some of the more complex topics taught in nursing programs, such as theory application and ethics. We commonly hear from students that these topics can be dry and lack engagement. We wanted to remedy this with a nontraditional approach to promote competency.

There is an increasing emphasis on change in the healthcare setting. We want MSN-prepared nurses to be ready to answer the call when change is needed. We want to crush the "way we have always done it" mentality because our stakeholders depend on us to produce excellence in practice and outcomes. We also wanted to provide a different perspective on the role of the nurse functioning within an interprofessional or interdisciplinary team, while providing tools that can be applied quickly.

We are passionate about the well-being of our profession and colleagues. We feel if we can teach our colleagues proper self-care strategies they are less likely to burn out and leave the profession. We teach caregivers of patients to take care of themselves, and we hope to remind nurses to do that for themselves as well.

We see this book supporting all nurses' transitions from the associate's degree or bachelor's degree preparation to the master's preparation. Irrespective of whether students reading this book have determined the path they would like to pursue, we believe the book will provide them a perspective of the various roles an MSN may hold and how each role works to support healthcare delivery.

Mindy Thompson
Brenda Scott

Acknowledgments

●●●●

We started this journey knowing that there was a gap in the literature on topics related to transitioning to master's degree nursing education and practice. Although we recognized the gap in resources, we did not have expertise in all areas of practice we wanted to include. We realized that we needed help to make this text a reality. We are grateful to the authors who have contributed to this book for joining us on this journey and for their contributions in shaping the future of nursing.

Many thanks to Springer Publishing Company for supporting us throughout this process and taking a chance on two first-time authors with a vision of writing something different from the usual nursing textbooks.

We thank our former faculty, particularly the NSU faculty, who never ceased to encourage and push us to the next level of excellence. Dr. Joyce VanNostrand, Dr. Diana Mashburn, and Dr. Jodi Gooden prepared us well for doctoral education and set high expectations for our professional achievements. And here we are—writing and publishing a textbook!

The most important acknowledgment for both of us to make is to God. Without Him, nothing is possible!

Brenda Scott
Mindy Thompson

First, I thank my brother, Brent, who is the second best nurse in my life (only after our mother). Not only have you challenged me to be the best nurse possible, but you made me an aunt. Thanks for providing three of life's greatest blessings, Bayli, Blayke, and Brylee. Although I may never be the parent or nurse that you are, I think I might have become smarter!

Next, Mindy Thompson deserves much gratitude. This textbook is published because you allowed me to pitch bold ideas and believed in me enough to chase dreams. I am honored to call you a friend and share this experience with you.

Mindy and I have been blessed with many mentors in our lives. A few of our former faculty members were acknowledged earlier, but there are a few other special teachers and professors I personally acknowledge for changing my life. First, Mrs. Cynthia Woods, my first-grade teacher at Dardanelle Elementary School. She is the reason I teach today. Thank you, Mrs. Woods, for believing in me and showing me how passion changes the lives of students. Second, I express much gratitude to Mrs. Lois Gotes. Thank you for always believing, "It'll be all right!" You demonstrated how a nursing instructor can care about a student while maintaining high expectations. Finally, many thanks to Dr. Arlene Hayne. Thank you for being a mentor and for encouraging me to slow down and soak in the experience. Your 30,000-foot perspective and "so, what" reflection has shaped my daily practice.

Family, friends, and esteemed colleagues, I express my gratitude to all of you for supporting me and making me the individual that I am today! I am so thankful that you are part of my cheering section. From my elementary, high school, and college friends, to the rowdy bunch in the ED, to the wacky health department crew, and all the amazing higher education teams, your expertise and practice guide me every day.

To all the individuals who have crossed or will cross my path, thank you for shaping my journey. I am eternally grateful to each of you!

Brenda Scott

To Scott: You have been my rock, even before I started nursing school! You have never complained once about the time I have spent in school or doing nursing-related activities. Any time I have ever asked for your thought on whether I should pursue a new interest, your answer is always the same: "If that's what you want to do…." You have always been there to remind me that I can do whatever I want to. I cannot express the full depth of my appreciation, admiration, and respect for you and the support you give me every day. I love you more than words and thank God for you every day.

To Aunt Sharon and Uncle Tom: I am so blessed to have your support. When nursing school seemed to be an opportunity that might not happen for me, you helped make sure it did. From taking care of me when I was little to taking care of Dakota when I went to college to start a career, you were always there to do whatever you could to ensure that I was successful. Thank you!

To Debi and Ronnie: You two have been a constant in our lives since I can remember. If I ever need some reminders of the faith mom had in me all I have to do is give you a call. You have the same faith in me as she had. You know that I am capable to do anything and are more than happy to remind me if needed. Making you proud is and has always been just as important to me as making mom proud. Debi, I am so glad to have you as a second mom!

To Robert and Vinita Carter: You know what you did and you know why I am thankful. Your actions will always be an inspiration to me!

Dr. Robin Harris: I am beyond thankful for you, your encouragement, and your guidance. You have modeled a great authentic leadership. You connect with people through your authenticity and show others how to use grace and humility. I am proud to know you and thankful to have you on my side.

Vega School District: I thank the amazing teachers I had in Vega, Texas. The names are many and the impact profound. From elementary to my final days as a senior, you all took a personal interest in each student's well-being and development. You were there to be more than a Math, Science, or English teacher: You were there to serve a purpose and to develop young people. Thank you for the time and energy you put into me. I am proud to be an alumnus of Vega High School and hope that Vega High School is equally proud of me.

Mindy Thompson

SECTION I

Foundations of Role Development in Master's-Level Nursing Education

Building a solid house depends on a good foundation; building the next step of your career also requires a strong base. In this section, we look at some historical perspectives, nursing theory, and ethics. When you think of nursing history, you probably either love it or not care so much. Either way, it is important to know where we came from to understand where we could go again if we are not careful. Pop Quiz: Who has a famous quote about that?* Now, another topic that most nurses usually dread is that of nursing theory. However, application of a theory is extremely important. You need to know how to select a theory that will fit various projects you are working on and appreciate why they are valuable in the process. We use the nursing process to explore and appreciate this skill. Finally, we break down ethics into a couple different components. We look at research ethics as well as bioethics. Until now, you may not have realized any differences in the field of ethics. There are entire books and courses on ethics, so we are going to keep things simple and give you the need to know versions in these areas.

---

*George Santayana (1863–1962): "Those who cannot remember the past are condemned to repeat it."

1

The History of Nursing

Nycole Oliver

OBJECTIVES

1. Identify important founders in nursing history.
2. Examine the actions of nursing historical figures that have influenced nursing today.
3. Identify nursing organizations that maintain the history of nursing.
4. Explore how the history of nursing influences current nursing practice.

The art of nursing has been in existence since the beginning of time. People have been caring for the ill and injured for as long as history has been recorded. In many early societies, no formal education for nurses was available, so the caregiver role was allocated to women, medicine men, shamans, or as predetermined by culture. The earliest nurses learned through traditions passed over generations, trial and error, as well as direct observation of other caregivers (Egenes, 2009).

The nursing profession was not identified as an organized career until the mid-1800s when Florence Nightingale cared for the sick and injured during the Crimean War. Since inception of nursing as a profession, several others have been instrumental in the development and evolvement of the role and have impacted how nursing is practiced today. The purpose of this chapter is to identify the founders of nursing, distinguish organizations maintaining the history of nursing, and discuss how the history of nursing influences modern nursing practice.

THE FOUNDERS OF NURSING

Numerous individuals contributed to major movements for nursing. Nightingale is probably the most well known and has been credited with laying the groundwork for the nursing profession. Countless others have been credited with key nursing advancements throughout the years. Along with nursing's founder, Nightingale, other nurses instrumental in building the foundation for nursing practice discussed in this section are the following: Dorothea Dix, Clara Barton, Linda Richards, and Lillian Wald.

Florence Nightingale

Nightingale, named after the city in which she was born, was born to a wealthy British family on May 12, 1820 (Whyte, 2010). As a child, she cared for sick people living in workers' cottages around her home. At a young age, she decided caring for people was her calling, a career that was ridiculed and considered a low-class profession at that time. Much to her parents' dismay, she trained with deaconesses and was soon appointed as superintendent of a small facility, the Upper Harley Street Hospital (Egenes, 2009; Whyte, 2010).

During the Crimean War in 1854, Nightingale learned the mortality rate for soldiers was almost 50%, from what she concluded was a result of poor living conditions. As a result, she gained permission to bring several ladies with her to the battlefields and introduced cleanliness and sanitation. Over the next several months, deaths and complications in the soldiers declined dramatically (Egenes, 2009). Although she was busy during the day caring for the sick and injured and immersed in administrative duties, she made time to visit soldiers at night, carrying a lamp to light her way. Her relentless compassion and caring while carrying her lamp gave rise to her nickname "The Lady With the Lamp." Nursing graduation ceremonies honor her memory by using lamps in their rituals (Stanley, 2007).

Nightingale documented the evidence-based care given and the decreased complications during the war and brought the information with her back to London. On her return to England in 1856, Nightingale raised money to fund the Nightingale School of Nursing at St. Thomas' Hospital in London for the education of professional nurses (Whyte, 2010). Students were educated in nursing theory and specialty care and were trained with clinical experiences on hospital wards (Egenes, 2009). Nightingale also authored the first nursing textbook, *Notes on Nursing*, in 1859 (Nightingale, 1859). Because of her significant contributions to nursing and healthcare in general, Nightingale's birthday is designated as National Nurses Day, with celebrations extending into the entire week. A pledge, written for Nightingale, called the Florence Nightingale Pledge, is also recited by new nurses before beginning to practice as a nurse.

Dorothea Dix

Dix, born in 1802, was known as a social reformer, and perhaps her most noted accomplishment is her efforts on behalf of the mentally ill. In the 1830s, she taught inmates at a prison in East Cambridge and was appalled at the living conditions in the prison. Both hardened criminals and mentally ill were housed together because at that time mental illness was not well understood. The mentally ill were not considered "ill," and a lot of times were removed from society and placed in cages or prisons. After witnessing the abysmal conditions the inmates lived in, she vowed to change things (Waldman, Rader, & Perlman, 2015).

Dix was appointed the Superintendent of Army Nurses during the Civil War in 1861. In the role, she was responsible for recruiting female nurses to care for sick and wounded soldiers. Nursing care for the soldiers improved significantly under her reign. Because of her tenacity and reputation for running a "tight ship," Dix obtained the nickname "Dragon Dix." After the war, she returned to her efforts regarding the mentally ill (Harshey-Meade, 2006; Waldman et al., 2015).

Over the course of the next half century, Dix lobbied for better living conditions for the mentally ill, fueling her passion with memories of the horrendous living conditions she observed while working in the prison before the war. Because of her tireless efforts, Dix changed the way people thought about the mentally ill, and mental hospitals were opened around the country to house the mentally ill and give them proper care (Waldman et al., 2015).

Clara Barton

Barton, born in 1821, started out as a teacher in her teen years. When the Civil War began in 1861, women were not permitted to serve on the battle-field, so Barton decided to care for soldiers in Washington City. At the time she did not have any formal training as a nurse, but still rallied to collect medical and other necessary supplies for soldiers on the battlefield. She quickly gained a reputation as an independent battlefield nurse, caring for soldiers from both armies. She was dubbed the "Angel of the Battlefield" by a surgeon during the war (Schmidt, 2004).

In 1863, Henry Dunant founded the International Red Cross to provide needed supplies and services during war. Many nations followed suit, signing the Geneva Treaty and forming separate national Red Cross organizations. The United States initially did not sign the treaty or form a Red Cross organization (Schmidt, 2004).

Barton traveled to Europe in 1869 and learned about the international Red Cross. She quickly saw the benefit of the organization, and on her return to the States in 1873, she campaigned and lobbied for the United States to support and form the American Red Cross to provide disaster relief to soldiers and their families. Several years later, in 1881, the American Association of the Red Cross was founded (now called the American Red Cross). Barton volunteered to serve as the first president of the organization (Schmidt, 2004).

Barton led the Red Cross for 23 years, and during her reign the organization handled numerous household and oversees disaster relief efforts. As a result of her efforts, the organization is still going strong today. The American Red Cross provides care for the victims of disasters in the form of international relief; blood collection, processing, and distribution; military and military family support; and training on health and safety (American Red Cross, 2018).

Linda Richards

Richards, born in 1841, is credited as "America's first trained nurse." She moved to Vermont as a child after her father's death and in her teens began informal training as a nurse. She cared for her mother as a young child, and for her ailing grandfather after her mother's death. At her grandfather's insistence, she went to school to become a teacher, but did not care for the teaching curriculum. When the Civil War began, she became very interested in the demand for nurses to care for soldiers and intrigued by reports of the women who cared for ill and injured soldiers in military hospitals. She had heard of the Nightingale School and Home for Nurses in London and wanted to pursue her dream of becoming a nurse (Holder, 2004; Munson, 1948).

In 1870, Richards decided to seek out learning opportunities for nursing inside a hospital. She moved to Boston and began working as an assistant nurse and ward maid at Boston City Hospital. She stayed for 3 months and left because of health issues. She then heard of a learning opportunity at the New England Hospital for Women and Children in Boston, where a training school for nurses would be opened. The school was taught by female physicians who were willing to train women as nurses. Richards enrolled in the training program in 1872 and graduated in 1873 (Holder, 2004; Munson, 1948).

Soon after graduation, Richards moved to New York and started teaching at Bellevue Hospital Training School, working closely with the nursing director to improve hospital conditions. She worked diligently as a patient advocate and lobbied for policy changes to enhance patient care. She even had the idea to keep a chart of patient records at the bedside so it was immediately available to others involved in the patient's care, a concept incorporated into such training programs as the Nightingale School of Nursing. She continued to advocate for formal nursing training and opened various schools of nursing, even as far away as Japan (Holder, 2004).

Lillian Wald

Wald, known as the "Mother of Public Health Nursing," was born to a wealthy German-Jewish family in Ohio in 1867 and moved to New York as a child. At the age of 16, she applied to Vassar College and was turned away because of her age. She watched a nurse take care of her older sister during childbirth and was so impressed that she convinced her parents to let her move to the city and pursue a nursing career. She was accepted into nursing school at the New York Hospital School of Nursing and graduated in 1891. On graduation, she began working at a juvenile asylum in Manhattan. Soon after, she decided to go to medical school (Ruel, 2014).

Shortly after beginning her studies in medical school, Wald observed both poverty and sickness in new refugees on the Lower East Side in Manhattan. The status of the refugees disgusted her so much that she dropped out of medical school and united with Mary Brewster, a fellow nurse, in moving into the illness and poverty-stricken neighborhood to care for immigrants in their homes. She soon realized health was only a small challenge faced by residents, and soon increased services to include teaching, offering arts, and assisting with career placement and housing (Henry Street Settlement, 2018; Ruel, 2014).

In 1893, the United States went through a major economic crisis, which prompted many new migrants to move from Ellis Island and into the city. Wald and Brewster formed the Henry Street Settlement and the Henry Street Visiting Nurse Service, now called the Visiting Nurse Service of

New York, which became the first and now the largest nonprofit home- and community-based health agency (Henry Street Settlement, 2018; Ruel, 2014).

A noted Jewish philanthropist, Jacob Schiff, was so impressed by Wald's work and organization that he gifted the organization a house at 265 Henry Street in 1895. For the next several years, the organization continued to grow and flourish, with Wald leading the way until 1933. During her time as a nursing pioneer, Wald also placed nurses in public schools and assisted with Columbia University School of Nursing's National Organization for Public Health Nursing (Henry Street Settlement, 2018).

Wald is remembered as a national leader in movements for public health, social reform, and human rights. Her relentlessness paid off, and her work is still in effect today. The Henry Street Settlement continues to serve the Lower East Side of Manhattan's population today through social services, arts, and healthcare programs. She even wrote a book, published in 1915, entitled *The House on Henry Street* (Henry Street Settlement, 2018).

ORGANIZATIONS MAINTAINING THE HISTORY OF NURSING

Along with standardized training for nurses, professional organizations are crucial for maintaining the profession and furthering patient care (Matthews, 2012). Since establishment of the profession, nurses have advocated for advancement of the role. As needs arose, organizations were founded to fill gaps between education and practice. Organizations discussed in this section are the following: National League for Nursing (NLN), American Nurses Association (ANA), and the International Council of Nurses.

National League for Nursing

After establishment of training programs for nurses, concerns were voiced regarding lack of educational standards. Training programs varied greatly in entrance requirements, curriculum, and length. In 1893, a national nursing organization was formed to address the concerns called the American Society of Superintendents of Training Schools of Nursing, later becoming the National League for Nursing Education, and eventually the NLN. The organization focuses on promoting standards for nursing education (Egenes, 2009).

The NLN advocates for a robust and diverse nursing workforce by endorsing distinction in nursing education. It purports the following core values: excellence, diversity, caring, and integrity. The organization offers networking opportunities, research grants, professional development, public policy initiatives, and testing services (NLN, n. d.).

American Nurses Association

In 1896, the Nurses' Associated Alumni of the United States and Canada was founded, and nearly 20 people attended the first convention. The association was later named the American Nurses Association (ANA) in 1911. The goal of the Association was to achieve licensure for nurses. States nurses' associations were formed as a result, and nurse practice acts for each state were eventually passed (ANA, 2018; Egenes, 2009).

Since the launch of the organization, the ANA has established a code of professional nursing, been involved in numerous publications regarding the nursing profession and nursing practice, become legislatively involved to advance the profession, and paved the way for registered nurses to be credentialed in specialty areas (ANA, 2018). After nurses were able to become credentialed in specialty areas, hundreds of national specialty organizations were established.

International Council of Nurses

In the late 1800s, the importance of networking between nurses of several nations was realized. In 1899, the International Council of Nurses was formed as the first international nursing organization. The mission of the organization is to represent nurses worldwide, influence health policy, and advance the profession. Core values include solidarity, accountability, visionary leadership, social justice, and innovativeness (International Council of Nurses, 2017).

HISTORY OF NURSING AS IT INFLUENCES MODERN PRACTICE

As discussed earlier, many of nursing's early pioneers have influenced modern practice. Nightingale laid the foundation for nursing practice and transformed it into the profession it is today. She changed the way people perceived nurses (drunken, disreputable, dishonest) into a trustworthy and honorable profession. Since 2001, according to the Gallup poll, the public has voted nursing as the most honest and ethical profession (Brenan, 2017).

Dix lobbied for improved care for the mentally ill, and her ideas have altered the perception of mental illness and given those who suffer from it the proper care they need. Barton lobbied to provide disaster relief nationwide, and her efforts are still in effect today. Richards saw the need for nursing training programs and led the way for nurses around the world to be properly educated in the field. Finally, Wald pioneered the public and community nursing movement, providing care for people and assisting with allocating available resources for people in the community.

Between the aforementioned innovators and many other early nurses' efforts, modern-day nursing would not be what it is today without the brave endeavors these women undertook. Nursing has grown as a profession and the people responsible for nursing as a reputable career have left their mark; their legacy will continue to be seeded in the occupation. This chapter has outlined some of the early founders of nursing, classified organizations maintaining the history of nursing, and examined how the history of nursing influences modern nursing practice.

CRITICAL THINKING QUESTIONS

1. In reviewing the founders of nursing discussed in this chapter, which founder do you relate to the most? Why?

2. What do you see as the role of the NLN, the ANA, and the International Council of Nurses in your practice as a master's-prepared nurse?

3. Why is your involvement in a national, state, or local nursing organization important?

4. Consider your current and future practice. How has history influenced what or how you practice?

5. Does new information about nursing history impact how you will practice nursing in the future? If yes, how? If not, why?

REFERENCES

American Red Cross. (2018). Founder Clara Barton. Retrieved from http://www.redcross.org/about-us/who-we-are/history/clara-barton

American Nurses Association. (2018). The history of the American Nurses Association. Retrieved from https://www.nursingworld.org/ana/about-ana/history/

Brenan, M. (2017, December 26). Americans rate nurses highest on honesty, ethical standards. *Gallup News*. Retrieved from news.gallup.com/poll/224639/nurses-keep-healthy-lead-honest-ethical-profession.aspx

Egenes, K. J. (2009). History of nursing. In G. Roux & J. A. Halstead (Eds.), *Issues and trends in nursing: Essential knowledge for today and tomorrow* (pp. 1–26). Sudbury, MA: Jones & Bartlett.

Harshey-Meade, G. (2006). Editors notes. Dorothea Dix: She was a nurse, advocate, and lobbyist. *Ohio Nurses Review, 81*(3), 6.

Henry Street Settlement. (2018). Retrieved from https://www.henrystreet.org

Holder, V. L. (2004). From handmaiden to right hand—the infancy of nursing. *AORN Journal, 79*(2), 374–382. doi:10.1016/S0001-2092(06)60614-5

International Council of Nurses. (2017). Our mission, strategic intent, core values, and priorities. Retrieved from http://www.icn.ch/who-we-are/our-mission-strategic-intent-core-values-and-priorities

Matthews, J. H. (2012). Role of professional organizations in advocating for the nursing profession. *Online Journal of Issues in Nursing, 17*(1), 3. doi:10.3912/OJIN.Vol17No01Man03

Munson, H. (1948). Linda Richards. *American Journal of Nursing, 48*(9), 551–555. doi:10.2307/3458627

National League for Nursing. (n. d.). Core values. Retrieved from http://www.nln.org/about/core-values

Nightingale, F. (1859). *Notes on nursing: What it is and what it is not.* London, UK: Harrison & Sons.

Ruel, S. R. (2014). Lillian Wald: A pioneer of home healthcare in the United States. *Home Healthcare Nurse, 32*(10), 597–600. doi:10.1097/NHH.0000000000000153

Schmidt, C. K. (2004). American Red Cross nursing: Essential to disaster relief. *American Journal of Nursing, 104*(8), 35–38. doi:10.1097/00000446-200408000-00025

Stanley, D. (2007). Lights in the shadows: Florence Nightingale and others who made their mark. *Contemporary Nurse, 24*(1), 45–51. doi:10.5555/conu.2007.24.1.45

Waldman, H. B., Rader, R., & Perlman, S. P. (2015). Healing "the most unkindest cut of all." *Exceptional Parent, 45*(12), 46–48.

Whyte, A. (2010). Relighting the lamp. *Nursing Standard, 24*(18), 18–20. doi:10.7748/ns.24.18.18.s25

CHAPTER 2

Nursing Process and Theory Selection

Mindy Thompson

OBJECTIVES

1. Recognize the importance of nursing theory.
2. Correlate the nursing process to theory application.
3. Evaluate a variety of theories as they apply to a concept.
4. Select a nursing theory to apply to a project.

Have you ever wondered why theories even matter? It is uncommon that you hear anyone sitting around talking about a specific theory. Theories are just for those academic types who do not have a life, right? Well, there is a little more to it than that. Theories are what provide a foundation for not only nursing practice but also research. Furthermore, theoretical frameworks can also help guide projects that may or may not have an actual research component. Theoretical or conceptual frameworks help provide direction to a project and can even help identify an outcome (Green, 2014). Of course, you may have seen research articles where no theory or framework was mentioned. Green (2014) argues that perhaps researchers are so comfortable with theories and frameworks they do not feel the need to explain them in the write-up of their study. As for the rest of us, keeping a theoretical or conceptual framework at the forefront of our project is very helpful.

Now, keep in mind, there are lots of types of theories out there. There are not only nursing theories that would guide direct patient care but also learning theories, systems theories, change theories, and many more. With so many kinds of theories, where in the world do you start to select one? In this chapter, we focus on using the nursing process to guide the selection of a theory for a project.

ASSESSMENT

As you know, the first step of the nursing process is assessment. So, logically, this is the first step of selecting a theory for your project. You will need to assess your project first. What type of project is it? Is your project aimed at direct patient care? Are you working in education? Are you looking to achieve a systems improvement? These questions will get you to the right category of theories to then begin narrowing your search.

For example, if you are doing a project in nursing education, you may want to look at teaching and learning theories. However, if your project is clinically based, a nursing theory may be better suited. Say, for instance, you are wanting to improve retention rates in a nursing program through the implementation of a program that will help students manage their stress and workload while in school. A nursing theory that may be used for this could be Dorothea Orem's Self-Care Theory or Sister Callista Roy's Adaptation Theory. Because this project example is not specific to the actual process of teaching and learning, a nursing theory may be better suited to allow consideration of the person as a whole. However, that is not to say a teaching or learning theory could not be used. If you are a nurse leader wanting to carry out a quality improvement project, choosing a systems theory or change theory would be more appropriate.

These are just a couple of quick examples that give you an idea of where to start in the assessment of your project to choose a theory. There are many categories of theories and it is not possible to list them all in this text; see Table 2.1 for some suggestions related to the roles for nurses with a master's degree identified by the American Association of Colleges of Nursing (AACN, 2011).

DIAGNOSE

Assuring you have an appropriate theory selected is much like deriving a nursing diagnosis. Now you have an idea of some of the categories of theories you can look for to align and guide your project. Next, you will want to assess the pairing to make sure they are a good fit to arrive at your final "diagnosis" or theory for the project. There are five components or tests to make sure your theory and project are a good match.

The first test of your theory "diagnosis" is logical congruence (Brathwaite, 2002). Logical congruence can be elaborately defined and explored, but to keep it simple: Does it make sense? Is it reasonable to say that the theory selected is applicable to the problem that exists in the project? Keep in mind that your project is aimed at solving some type of problem. So, is the theory

TABLE 2.1 AACN Master's Roles and Possible Theoretical Categories

	ROLE	THEORETICAL CATEGORY
Direct Care Roles	Clinical Nurse Leader	Systems, Organizational, Change, Behavioral, Leadership
	Educator	Teaching, Learning, Systems, Change, Behavioral, Nursing
	Advanced Practice	Nursing, Change, Behavioral
Indirect Care Roles	Public Health Nurse	Nursing, Change, Behavioral, Systems
	Informaticist	Systems, Organizational, Change
	Clinical Research Coordinator	Nursing, Change, Behavioral, Systems
	Nurse Administrator	Systems, Organizational, Change, Behavioral, Leadership

AACN, American Association of Colleges of Nursing.

selected operating on the same viewpoints you have about your project? If so, it has passed step one of diagnosis.

The second test is conceptual clarity. This term refers to the direct association of relational statements within the theory as well as the project that show the two are associated or there is some causality between the two (Brathwaite, 2002). A project was mentioned earlier in which focusing on student retention may result in using the Self-Care Theory or Adaptation Theory if the project is focused on stress management of the student. The theories of Self-Care and Adaptation fit conceptually because the project is focused on stress management. If the posed intervention for the retention problem was more related to an action focused on a change to the program itself rather than the student, a systems theory or organizational theory may be better suited. Do you see how these two concepts differ?

The third test is to evaluate the level of abstraction that can range from concrete to abstract (Brathwaite, 2002). A concrete level theory will be a direct and linear explanation of how the theory explains or relates to the project. When working with a theory that has a concrete level of abstraction, outcomes often form naturally when applying the theory to the project as they are directly measurable (Walker & Avant, 2010). On the contrary, highly abstract levels of theory are often referred to as middle range or grand theories and are not limited by time or space nor are they directly measurable (Brathwaite, 2002).

Although there are many grand theories used to guide nursing projects, these are conceptual and provide key concepts and principles to the discipline as a whole. Some examples of these are Roy's Adaptation Theory or Watson's Theory of Caring. A middle-range theory is more specific but only dissects a situation with a limited number of variables. Examples of middle-range nursing theories include Lenz and Pugh's Theory of Unpleasant Symptoms and Mishel's Uncertainty of Illness Theory. In addition, there is practice theory that looks at a specific nursing situation and identifies explicit goals as well as how those goals will be met. A couple of examples of practice theory are Neuman's System Model and Peplau's Interpersonal Theory.

The fourth test is that of clinical utility. Does the theoretical model you are considering apply to practice in the real world? The model chosen should help explain either the problem being resolved by the project or the intervention needed to solve the problem (Brathwaite, 2002). If this is true of the model being considered, there is potential to influence nursing practice and the model would be considered a good fit or a proper "diagnosis."

The last component to consider is cultural competence (Brathwaite, 2002). Cultural competence is a concept that is difficult to measure (Loftin, Hartin, Branson, & Reyes, 2013). However, it is one that clinicians are believed to have superior knowledge compared with the clients they serve (Brathwaite, 2002). In terms of selecting a theory for a project, a theory should allow for cultural sensitivity for the client served and to further support a clinician's cultural competence.

PLAN AND IMPLEMENT

Now that you have selected a theory believed to align with your project, the next step is to plan your project using your theory as a guide. Nursing theories are essentially an explanation of the nursing process, so they are a logical source to help you lay out your project. Now, it would be wonderful if theories were laid out like a standardized care plan and gave you step-by-step options to apply to your specific project. Although it is not quite that simple, it is not necessarily difficult either. There is a plethora of locations to learn about different theories from textbooks to websites.

Whatever source you use to learn about your theory, you need to look for the major components. These typically include categories such as assumptions, major concepts, strengths, and weaknesses. Let us look at the theory of cybernetics and see how it would be used to plan a project.

The first major concept of cybernetics is that it introduces the concept of circularity and circular causal systems (Heims, 1980). This concept equates to a process being repetitive or circular in function—just like the nursing process! Simply, you complete a cycle of steps and the process repeats over and over again. So, in planning your project, you have probably already identified a process that is circular or repetitive in nature and this trait may have been one reason you picked this theory in the first place.

The second major concept of cybernetics is that systems within the project are defined by boundaries (Heims, 1980). Say, for instance, you are doing a project that involves different departments to create interprofessional collaboration. Each discipline is defined by boundaries or scopes of practice in which they work (Heims, 1980). Along this same line, the next major concept is the notion that every system has a goal (Heims, 1980). Although each discipline of an interdisciplinary team may be working toward common patient care goals of safety and quality, each has its own discipline-specific goal (Heims, 1980). In addition, each system acts in accordance to achieve the goal (Heims, 1980). In planning your project with this theory, you would consider the disciplines or systems that are impacting what you are trying to change. Are there multiple disciplines impacting the outcome? Are there different systems, such as a network and processes, that are influencing that in which you are trying to make a change? If so, incorporate these different components into your plan to provide direction.

The next major concept of this theory states that the environment affects the aim (Heims, 1980). For instance, if you are working on a systems-related issue in informatics, the direction of the project is dependent on a few environmental conditions. Some of these may include the literal environment of the network that could do physical harm or the political environment that may or may not support the project. Either way or for any project, you would need a supportive environment for the project. In planning your project, is there anything in the environment that you would need to address as part of your plan? If so, write that up as part of your plan. If not, you can address how environmental conditions are controlled and move on with the theory.

The next major concept to consider in your plan is how information will flow through the circular process providing feedback as the project progresses (Heims, 1980). What information will you need to collect? What information will be meaningful to evaluate your project? What information may inform future versions of the process your project proposes? Whenever a project is implemented, there are often things learned along the way that create ideas for improvements to the initial plan. Making changes to the plan in the midst of implementation should not be done, but addressing new ideas gleaned from information in the implementation process should be included in the conclusion piece of the project.

Another major concept of the cybernetics theory is that the system measures the difference between the current state and the goal to be achieved (Heims, 1980). When planning your project, this measure would be a good piece of the theory to use in guiding your evaluation plan as it is an evaluative statement. The piece to focus on is whether the measurement is coming from the system itself. In looking at your particular project, what is your system? Is it an interdisciplinary team? Is it a patient population? Is it an academic issue where the system is a course or maybe even the whole program?

The next major concept of the cybernetics theory is that the system will detect errors and will take corrective action to remain focused on the goal (Heims, 1980). Now, these concepts are not as easy to directly correlate to a nursing project. However, the body detecting errors and taking corrective actions to maintain homeostasis is a good example. Again, think about your specific project. Perhaps your project is something you have created, such as an automatic response to an event, For instance, in an educational setting where students take online examinations, you have devised a plan for a learning management system to send an auto-generated response to a student on the basis of a particular examination score. This theory would help you identify a step in your project plan to assure that the system can detect an error and do something to correct it or signal a need for correction should an error occur.

The cybernetics theory is just one randomly selected theory used to help illustrate how you would use a theory to help plan a project. Although the theory was randomly selected, it was selected as a non-nursing theory and one not routinely seen in the nursing literature. However, it is a good illustration of how almost any theory could be used as long as it fits your project's concepts and goals. Do not be afraid to think beyond the obvious for that is where innovation lives.

EVALUATE

Just like when you write a nursing care plan and the outcome is the positive spin-off of the nursing diagnosis, the overall outcome of your project is the solution you hope to see to address the problem you have identified. However, you do need objective statements that lead you to the identified outcome. In addition, just like in a nursing care plan, your objective statements determine how you will evaluate your project. Because you built your project with a theoretical framework, your evaluation methods will also be theoretically based. It is important to develop a clear evaluation plan before beginning your project. This plan helps you identify what is successful and what needs revisions.

At first glance, and maybe the second or third, selecting and applying a theory to a project may feel quite overwhelming or even confusing. Remember to think of the theory as a guide. You are looking for a structure to align your project so that you can make sure you are considering as many components as possible and addressing the identified problem thoroughly. The nursing process is an excellent framework to solve almost any problem and you already know it well. Use what you know and the strengths you have to build new skills or expand ones you already possess.

CRITICAL THINKING QUESTIONS

1. Select a nursing theory. Discuss how this theory either does or does not support culturally competent care.

2. Consider your daily practice. Discuss a nursing theory that aligns with how you view your practice as a nurse. What do you do that aligns with the theory's assumptions?

3. Make a table of three nursing theories that could be applied to your project. Be sure to include the theory's assumptions, limitations, and how it correlates to your project.

4. Explain the pros and cons of using a grand theory, a midrange theory, or a practice theory.

5. Select a non-nursing theory. Consider how this theory could be used to address a nursing problem. What additional ways could you use this theory to support a project?

REFERENCES

American Association of Colleges of Nursing. (2011). The essentials of master's education in nursing. Retrieved from http://www.aacnnursing.org/Education-Resources/AACN-Essentials

Brathwaite, A. (2002). Selection of a conceptual model framework for guiding research interventions. *Internet Journal of Advanced Nursing Practice*, 6(1), 1–8. Retrieved from https://print.ispub.com/api/0/ispub-article/8576

Green, H. E. (2014). Use of theoretical and conceptual frameworks in qualitative research. *Nurse Researcher, 21*(6), 34–38. doi:10.7748/nr.21.6.34.e1252

Heims, S. J. (1980). *John von Neumann and Norbert Wiener: From mathematics to the technologies of life and death.* Cambridge, MA: MIT Press.

Loftin, C., Hartin, V., Branson, M., & Reyes, H. (2013). Measures of cultural competence in nurses: An integrative review. *Scientific World Journal, 2013,* 289101. doi:10.1155/2013/289101

Olszewski Walker, L., & Coalson Avant, K. (2010). *Strategies for theory construction in nursing* (5th ed.). London, UK: Pearson.

3

Ethics in Nursing Research

Tara Slagle

OBJECTIVES

1. Identify basic concepts of ethics.
2. Explore how beneficence, justice, and respect influence research.
3. Discuss historical events that guide research.
4. Examine methods for the protection of human subjects.

As you develop your role as a master's-prepared nurse (MSN), you will come across the topic of ethics in nursing research. Ethics is a topic that is important to revisit at each level of a nurse's education. Basic terms are defined and discussed in undergraduate courses and the introduction of nursing research will always include a discussion on research ethics. Once you step into the advanced role of an MSN, irrespective of whether you ask for it, you will gain more responsibility. Responsibilities include setting an example for other nurses, responsibility of thinking through a problem versus reactively answering it, and the responsibility of knowing when an ethical issue arises and having to ask the hard questions.

I know nursing research may not be at the top of your list when it comes to favorite subjects. And even more so, ethics in nursing research probably has you falling asleep before you finish this sentence. I am here to tell you that nursing research is daunting. However, this is where change is made. Nursing research is where nursing is growing vastly and is raising the bar of the profession of nursing. The role of ethics in nursing must be understood to completely understand the role of nursing in research. To frame the role of ethics in nursing research, I think it is important to discuss examples of ethics in nursing and how your current experiences apply to ethics in the context of nursing research.

CURRENT PRESENCE OF ETHICS IN NURSING

At this point in your nursing career, I am sure that you have heard the term ethics. Ethics may mean a multitude of different things to each and every one of you. For example, if you work or have worked in an intensive care unit (ICU), you may have dealt with ethics while caring for a patient who was on life support and decisions needed to be made about the future of that patient. For example, the patient has a signed do not resuscitate (DNR) order, but the family has chosen to keep him or her alive. If you work or have worked in maternity, you may have dealt with a multitude of scenarios from a mother who used drugs to birth of a child with a low probability of survival. In 2017, Alex Wubles, an emergency room nurse in Utah, was following ethical policies in refusing to draw blood from an unconscious patient and was even threatened and handcuffed by a police officer for upholding an ethical decision in the name of her patient (Wamsley, 2017). I am going to make the assumption that every nurse has dealt with or has been a part of an ethical decision-making process whether he or she knew it at the time.

In our daily nursing practice, we abide by the laws of our license, laws of the government, guidelines of our policies, and what we are told to do. When we discuss ethics, we are many times discussing the dreaded gray areas, the areas where the hard decisions need to be made. These decisions are hard because they may conflict with our own beliefs or may conflict with what we think is morally right. As nurses, we must uphold the ethical principles by our patients' rights. The nursing Code of Ethics has been established by the American Nurses Association (ANA). The code includes important concepts that guide nurses when gray areas occur. The difficult thing about the ANA's code of ethics is sometimes interpreting the code. Nurses many times use a support team from their facility to help make ethical decisions. In most all healthcare organizations, there is a required ethical team. This team is called the institutional review board (IRB). We discuss the IRB in more detail later.

RESEARCH ETHICS

Now that we covered a basic overview of ethics in nursing, we can now discuss the role of ethics in nursing research. The terms that you need to know as the basic backbones of ethics are beneficence, justice, respect for persons, and nonmaleficence. These are the terms you learned in Ethics 101, but when related to the professional role of the MSN, they become real-world tools used to make decisions. These terms are defined and discussed in the context of their presence in nursing research ethics.

Beneficence

Beneficence is better known as the doctor's code: "Do no harm." When conducting research, the goal is to not harm the participants first and foremost, followed by the research results themselves. Let me share an example and you tell me if you think this research proposal follows the ethical principle of beneficence.

VIGNETTE 3.1

Your facility is having an issue with a sudden increase in falls. Your team discusses many options and finds a new alarm device that you agree would be a great option for your patients. The alarms are expensive and at this time you can afford to have enough for only half of your residents. Your team is very excited for the expectation of a drastic decrease in falls, so you choose to complete a research study on the alarms and fall rates so that you can show your shareholders the worth of the alarms and convince them to buy all patients these alarms. You decide that you want to conduct a quasiexperimental study where you do not randomly assign patient participants; they are assigned on the basis of which hallway their rooms are located on. You have one hallway of patients with the new fall prevention alarms (intervention group) and the other hallway with no alarms (control group) so you can see if your new alarms prevent falls.

This appears to be a great study; you want to prevent falls and you also want to complete this study so you can share your findings with other facilities on the wonderful results you had. Before you start the study, does this proposal follow the ethical principle of beneficence?

No. This is not a study that follows the ethical principle of beneficence. This study could cause more harm than good, and it would not be approved through IRB. What is wrong?

Answer: You are taking away a current safety mechanism for the control group. Patients who are at risk of falling and who are in the control group are not being allowed to have alarms and therefore any of them could fall and harm could occur. As the researcher, you would reorganize your study, and now your control group will have their current alarms in place, while the intervention group will have the new alarms. Your study will now be approved and safe because you are not taking away from the control group.

Justice

Justice in ethics is the inclusion of fairness. Justice is discussed in the environment of participant selection. Many researchers account for the inclusion of justice by basing their participants' selection on a randomized process such as a blind study where participants are assigned a number randomly and the researcher picks a set of numbers not ever knowing which participants correlate to those numbers.

The other side of justice in research is the right to fair treatment with equal dissemination of benefit and burden. Think about the recruitment tactics that are used in research. You need participants in your research study, but people are busy and many times want to be compensated for their time. Knowing this as a researcher, the thought may be to recruit individuals who have a lower socioeconomic status as they would be assumed to be more motivated. This preconception could be considered injustice if the benefits of the study are not a benefit to those of lower socioeconomic status.

VIGNETTE 3.2

In the Muslim culture, a baby is breastfed by its mother or wet nurse until the age of 2 years. The nurse researcher goes to an area with a high Muslim population but low socioeconomic status and offers money for participation in a research study about the progression of weight of children who breastfeed and progression of weight of children who do not breastfeed. The study would include that by random selection some mothers would be asked to withhold breastfeeding and would be given formula to supplement. Does this proposal follow justice?

No. This is not a study that follows the ethical principle of justice. This study could cause more harm than good, and it would not be approved through IRB. What is wrong?

Answer: The participant selection of low socioeconomic participants was chosen to increase the researcher's ability to gain participants with the offer of money. The researcher was asking participants to choose between their religious practices of breastfeeding and money that they may need to survive.

Respect for Persons

This ethical principle is very well known to nurses as informed consent. The informed consent allows the participants the ability to be educated and to make their own decisions on what happens to them or any risks or benefits that may occur to them on the basis of their decision.

As nurses, we may see this process as obtaining a signature, but knowing what it truly means is an important reminder. The informed consent is a verification of a discussion. The verification must include the action to be performed, the benefits of the action, and the risks. The participant must be given clear direction on how to ask questions. The agreement made verifies that all matters on the consent were addressed and both parties are aware and in agreement.

In the context of nursing research, respect for persons is a process within itself. During the proposal stage of a research study, the informed consent will be developed. All of the ethical principles we have discussed will need to be evaluated in the informed consent. Once the informed consent is developed, it will be brought before the IRB along with any additional documents such as the recruitment script. The IRB will review and evaluate the consent to be sure that all areas of the study are communicated. The communication of an informed consent is even evaluated to be sure that it is written at a fifth-grade reading level.

VIGNETTE 3.3

As the researcher, you develop your informed consent. You have chosen to complete a study on bedside shift report and whether it is effective in increasing patient satisfaction. The participants in the study will complete bedside shift report for a period of time and patient satisfaction scores will be measured to see if there is a correlation. What the participant does not know is that the nursing leadership team will be listening outside of the doors of some of the staff so they can verify that the report is being given correctly. The researcher did not want to reveal this information as he or she was afraid that the students would be biased. This bias is known as the Hawthorne effect and is addressed in the section "Hawthorne Effect." Does this consent follow respect for persons?

No. This is not a study that follows the ethical principle of respect for persons. This study could cause more harm than good, and it would not be approved through IRB. What is wrong?

Answer: This omission of the risk of leadership in monitoring participants in this study keeps the informed consent from being ethical. It is not to say that all informed consent must always reveal every aspect of studies, but in this case the benefit does not outweigh the risk. The participants could choose to not follow the bedside shift report while a leader was monitoring them, and this noncompliant could have a direct effect on how that leader sees this employee. The effect could show up on the performance evaluation of the employee or could be used against the employee when an opportunity arises such as a promotion. There are other options such as including the possibility of leadership listed on the consent, although the participants may not know when, or having those who listen in be staff nurses who have no influence on the participants' evaluation.

Research Ethics in the History of Medicine

We are going to assume goodwill as we discuss research ethics throughout history. Researchers spend a lot of time testing their hypotheses and become very committed to their studies. Imagine being the researcher who someday cures cancer; he or she may spend his or her whole life testing hypothesis after hypothesis, motivated by the idea of saving millions of lives. Throughout his or her process, he or she may have an idea that he or she wants to test, but once he or she applies for ethical approval, he or she is turned down because the test subjects are seen at higher risk than the possible benefit. This scenario occurs often, and therefore the discussion of ethics and the IRBs is in place. There must be checks and balances, even when the research is developed with the best of intentions. This does not mean that studies are cancelled; it means that the researchers need to develop a different study, one that is less to no risk until it can show some proven benefit that outweighs the risk.

HISTORICAL PERSPECTIVES

I truly do not feel that I can discuss research ethics without including a history lesson. History is important in the topic of ethics because as humans we must always learn from the past. We must understand what occurred so we can be sure to not repeat these tragedies.

Nuremberg

In 1947, the Nuremberg Code was established as a result of the heinous human experimentation used by Nazi physicians in concentration camps. The trials that occurred are a story in themselves, but I am discussing the code and how it affects human research today. Many of the experiments that were done did not include any type of informed consent, and the ones that may have had consent used coercion to obtain it. This aspect of consent is the focus of our discussion on the Nuremberg Code. It is easy enough to say that researchers will obtain consent, but how that consent is obtained is very important.

Informed consents must enclose all details of a study to include the purpose of the research, the procedures to be followed, and many risks that the participants may have if they participate. Confidentiality is an important component and requires an explanation of how it will be kept. Participants must also be given the option of leaving the study at any time of their own free will. The Nuremberg Code specifically states that the voluntary consent of the human subject is essential. Many excuses were used in the Nuremberg trials, but the code also defines that research done in the name of the greater good but infringing on the rights of individuals is not acceptable.

Tuskegee

A Public Health Service (PHS) study was started in Tuskegee, Alabama, in 1932. The study was an effort by the PHS to prove the need for treatment of syphilis with a focus on African American populations. A total of 600 black men participated in the study and were told that they were a part of a study where they were being treated for "bad blood" and that included them receiving free health checkups, free meals, and burial insurance (Centers for Disease Control and Prevention [CDC], 2017).

In July 1972, a news article was published revealed that these men were never given an informed consent and in fact they were purposefully not being treated for syphilis so researchers could show the progression of the disease if not treated. As I mentioned earlier, we start by assuming goodwill in knowing that the researchers felt they were doing a good thing in learning about a disease and allowing it to progress so they could argue the need for clinics and funds to help treat syphilis. In this study, however, they sacrificed the health of their participants; that is not ethically or morally just. This study was ended in 1972, after it had gone on for 40 years.

This study was groundbreaking for researchers and research ethics. The program was taken over by the CDC. In 1974, the National Research Act was enacted and defined essential components of ethical research practices. Voluntary consent is now required of research participants in studies funded by the Department of Health and Human Services and an institutional review board (IRB) must always review any research dealing with human subjects.

ETHICS IN MSN NURSING

Wow, we have covered a lot of ground on the subject of ethics. I am sure you are now asking yourself: What does this mean to me? I remember my own journey in the role of an MSN. I had decided to follow the path of nursing education because I wanted to give back to the nursing profession and I wanted to be like the amazing nursing instructors that I had, the ones who not only taught me what I needed to know to pass the NCLEX® but also taught me how to be compassionate and caring and to always put the patient first. Through the educational journey, I worked as a night-shift bedside nurse in an emergency department (ED). I spent some evenings writing papers and studying around 3 a.m., if we were lucky enough to have a lull. I was absorbing so much information it was hard to tell which things were going to help me as an educator.

I can now tell you that it all matters. As an educator, I have taught all the things I learned and not only had to define the terms and know what they are but also had to absorb the knowledge and then convert it into what will motivate my students and what will make them want to care about nursing theory or public health or ethics. The greatest tool an educator can have is experience. Being able to experience the development of a new nursing theory and then see its influence on the profession make a dry subject turn into a passion. My own experiences with nursing research and ethics within nursing research have allowed me the ability to say that I am passionate about this subject, and I hope that shines through in this chapter.

So enough about my journey, why does nursing research ethics matter to you? My hope is that many of you will consider continuing your education even beyond the master's level into the doctorate level. With great power comes great responsibility, and nursing truly encompasses this saying. The inclusion of evidence-based practice in nursing has allowed for an increase in collegial discussion among nurses and physicians. Nurses are no longer the task doers for physicians; we are practitioners of nursing care and what we do, we do because we know it is the best for those in our care. Defining nursing as its own profession is still a constant battle, but our armor and our defense is research. The ability to read research, know its strength, and translate its meaning allows nurses to advocate even more strongly for our best practices.

Once you are in the habit of reading and translating research, you can then begin to enact experiments. These experiments may be evidence-based practice studies, original research, or even quality projects. Many times, when working at the bedside, nurses begin with quality projects on the basis of evidence-based best practices.

For example, there are numerous studies that support different variations of sepsis screenings. These screening tools have been shown to alert healthcare staff to patients who have sepsis or are at high risk for sepsis. These screenings can be implemented into practice and a quality study can be done to see whether they truly support early recognition of sepsis. Knowing that the treatment of sepsis includes early antibiotics, fluids, and monitoring of lactic acid levels, these screenings could essentially save lives. Although many quality projects do not require IRB approval, a diligent nurse would think through the implementation of this screening to be sure to eliminate any risk to patients.

Another example is with simulation. Many facilities use simulation as an ideal tool to provide experience and education to nurses. There is no IRB approval required to conduct a simulation, but it still cannot hurt to think through ethical principles. If a simulation of a cardiac arrest is held on a nursing unit during their busiest time and during a shift that has limited staffing, will the other patients be at increased risk? There may be a multitude of different options and maybe no true answer to this question, but what can you do as the nurse who now knows about ethics to mitigate any harm or risk to the other patients while the simulation is occurring? Can you ask additional staff to be on hand to support the other patients while the simulation occurs? Can you be open to cancelling or postponing the simulation if the environment is unsafe? All of these questions are great questions to ask yourself as an MSN. You can no longer see things as black and white, but as opportunities to see multiple answers and multiple options.

Research ethics truly applies to the ethical considerations taken when research is conducted, but the knowledge that ethics brings can be applicable in multiple situations. Quality studies are the most relatable studies that many nurses are involved in almost daily. Through experiencing these studies and relating them to research, you can grow in your ethical knowledge as well as knowledge into evidence-based practice and nursing research. One interesting research term to think about when being involved in any type of quality evidence-based practice or original research study is the Hawthorne effect.

Hawthorne Effect

The Hawthorne effect originated in a factory near Chicago in Hawthorne. The factory workers were more productive when they were being observed by their supervisors during a research study than when they were working under normal conditions. With the important and essential inclusion of informed consent, the idea is that when participants know that they are being monitored, they are more likely to follow the rules and be top performers than if they were working in the business as usual environment.

STRATEGIES TO ENSURE HUMAN SUBJECTS' RIGHTS ARE PROTECTED

Federal Guidelines

The federal government has guidelines for protecting human rights during research through the Belmont Report (BR). The BR was developed from the 1974 National Research Act. The report was one of the requirements of the act that basic components of ethics would be defined and outlined as guidelines for researchers to follow. The report is used by IRBs when they are asked to review research proposals. The three major headings in the BR are boundaries between practice and research, basic ethical principles, and research applications (Department of Health and Human Services, 2017). Within these three sections of the report are three principles that you should know well by now because you just read about them earlier in this chapter: respect for persons, beneficence, and justice. Ethics is many times seen as subjective and, irrespective of whether you agree with this, it is hopefully understood that having guidelines to making decisions in ethics is essential. The BR brings each IRB a set of guidelines to aid in making a decision. These guidelines also brings to light the fact that an IRB is not one person but a group of persons who approve research. Many of us have different personal values and principles, so it only helps an IRB to include multiple people to bring different viewpoints to the hypothetical table.

For example, the BR discusses in its chapter on respect for persons the importance of people being given choices and options. No one should ever feel forced to participate in a research study. A research recruiter can explain and try to encourage participation but at the end of the day it is each individual's choice to participate or not. The second part of respect for persons includes the discussion on those with impaired decision-making abilities, such as people who are in prison, children, or even pregnant women. In nursing, we know these to be vulnerable populations, and this holds true in research. We must protect these individuals by giving them even more choices and options. For example, we must be mindful of the consequences of offering monetary gifts for participation to a mother who may be struggling with an inability to support her newborn child.

The second principle of the BR discusses beneficence that, as discussed earlier, is the essential do no harm. The researchers must take all measures possible to reduce any possible harm from coming to participants. The researchers must also clearly outline for participants any risks they may be taking even if all possible measures have been taken to decrease risks in the informed consent, so a participant can choose to not participate if he or she does not want to take that risk. For example, your nursing council decides to complete a study on lateral violence and sends out an anonymous survey asking nurses whether they have ever participated in lateral violence against a coworker. Right away you would ask whether these nurses would be honest, but truly the real question is: How can you protect the nurses so that they feel safe being honest? In this example, as researchers, we would thoughtfully lay out step by the step the ways we would guarantee that the results of the study could not be traced back to an individual nurse. First off, the researchers cannot be anyone who has any authority over the nurses or their performance evaluations. Second, a third-party site would be used to collect the data so that there would be no way to trace an email address or handwriting. Third, the demographic data would not be used if these lead to the identification of an individual, for example, if there is only one man who works in a particular department. Finally, you would identify who will have access to the online survey login and what will occur with the data after the study is over. The data must be kept for 7 years in a password-locked device and then destroyed after 7 years. There could very well be more ways to show protection and these can be seen as the minimum way to maximize benefits and minimize harm.

The third principle of the IRB is justice. Justice refers to being fair and equal. It includes consent, inclusion criteria, and exclusion criteria. The IRB must be sure that participants are selected on the basis of merit and not just because a specific person or population is easy to access. A great example is the use of research in prisons. We already discussed how prisoners are vulnerable populations, so they receive increased protection. If I wanted to research favorite colors, it may seem easy to use prisoners because they are in a contained space and may be assumed to be easy to obtain feedback from; however, prison demographics do not represent the greater demographics of the country. Therefore, if you want to know the favorite color of the people of America, prisoners are not the best population to use.

Organizational Guidelines

Individual organizations use the federal guidelines of the BR to make decisions in their individual IRBs. Having an IRB is a social responsibility of individual organizations. Most hospitals and schools are required to have an ethics committee. In 1992, The Joint Commission required that hospitals have a forum for discussing ethical issues. Does your facility have an ethics committee? Who is on it? If you do not already know, it can be fascinating to ask and see. My facility has an ethics committee that consists of a social worker, chaplain, human resources representative, and a medical director.

CASE STUDY

What kind of nursing educator would I be if I did not include a case study at least once? Following is an example of a research proposal. Once you have read through the proposal, take a moment to think through everything you have just read and consider the three principles of the BR to determine whether the human subject rights have been protected.

During the most recent steering council meeting, the ED nurses were discussing the recent increased census and the increase in the number of nurses who were calling out sick and working overtime. The chair of the council shared that he had read a recent article on the effects of mindfulness activities to reduce stress in post–open-heart surgery patients. The chair proceeded to discuss a thought that maybe the nursing staff could benefit from mindfulness training and that the topic could be a great research study for the upcoming Magnet® redesignation.

The proposed study was developed and read as follows:

Study: Determining the effect of mindfulness training on nurses' overall stress. Half of the nurses will be randomly sent to a 4-hour mindfulness training session. The nurses who attend the mindfulness study will be recorded and their surveys will be separated out into an intervention group. The nurses who do not participate in the education will be placed in a control group.

Setting: Three EDs within a three-campus hospital system. A total of 250 nurses are employed in the ED.

Data collection procedures: A survey link will be emailed to all the nurses in the three EDs. The lead researcher will be the only one with access to the survey results and the lead researcher is the educator for one of the departments but has no authority on staff performance evaluations. The informed consent will be included on the first page of the survey and will include any and all risks or benefits of the study. The participants must agree to the informed consent to move forward in the survey. The survey will include an overall health assessment using a valid and reliable instrument. A posttest will be sent out 1 month later asking the same questions.

Requirements of participants: *Voluntary participation in the survey. Survey participation includes agreeing or disagreeing to an informed consent and completion of both a pretest and a posttest survey.*

Risks/benefits: The participants will not be at any risk with participation and will not receive any benefits.

After reviewing the above-stated proposal, put yourself in the role of a member of the IRB. Would you approve this study as is?

How does the proposal meet respect for persons?

How does the study meet beneficence?

How does the study meet justice?

Answer: This study is off to a good start, but the staff have not been diligent in including everything needed.

Respect for persons: The study does not explain how confidentiality will be kept. Because there are two groups of nurses and those in the mindfulness classes will be named, how will the researchers know which surveys are theirs? Researchers tend to use a code to define who is who while also keeping confidentiality. For example, the students can use the last four digits of their phone number when completing the survey and also when signing into the educational session.

Beneficence: The study does not appear to do any harm; however, there are possible benefits to those who participate in the education, if it is seen as a positive intervention. The researchers should discuss how they can offer the education to everyone after the study is completed as to not withhold a positive experience from nurses who could benefit.

Justice: Justice has been kept with including an informed consent; however, the researchers must include the benefits of the education and the upfront risks of not having the education to the participants as well as a discussion on confidentiality for the consent to be thorough.

Human subject protection is truly simple in its basic design to respect individuals, cause no harm, and provide equal opportunities. The gray areas of this statement include the ability of giving options and choices and protecting those who are vulnerable. To many nurses this is something we do on a daily basis, but we should also understand the importance in following ethical guidelines and always being thorough in participation in and conducting research in terms of human subject protection.

CRITICAL THINKING QUESTIONS

1. Discuss examples of what you do in your current nursing practice to embody ethical principles of beneficence, justice, and respect for persons.

2. Nuremberg and Tuskegee obviously had long-term impacts on the field of research. Discuss the role and importance of IRBs.

3. Conduct a resource search on the Hawthorne effect. What do you think? Myth or truth? Justify your opinion with scholarly and credible sources.

4. Research organizational guidelines for the institution or organization where you plan to complete your capstone project. How will you incorporate protection of human rights into your project?

REFERENCES

Centers for Disease Control and Prevention. (2017). The Tuskegee Timeline. Retrieved from https://www.cdc.gov/tuskegee/timeline.htm

Department of Health and Human Services. (2017). The Belmont Report: Ethical principles and guidelines for the protection of human subjects of research. Retrieved from https://www.hhs.gov/ohrp/regulations-and-policy/belmont-report/index.html

Wamsley, L. (2017). Utah nurse arrested for doing her job reaches $500,000 settlement [blog post]. *National Public Radio*. Retrieved from https://www.npr.org/sections/thetwo-way/2017/11/01/561337106/utah-nurse-arrested-for-doing-her-job-reaches-500-000-settlement

4 •••••

Clinical Ethics and the Role of the MSN

Lea Brandt and Lori Popejoy

OBJECTIVES

1. Define clinical ethics as it applies to the role of the nurses with master's degrees.
2. Differentiate between ethics, morality, and the law.
3. Appreciate the role of ethical and legal principles in bioethics.
4. Identify strategies that promote ethical practice.

Most nurses practice ethics every day without realizing they are applying the concepts of *right* and *wrong* to choices in their professional lives. The study of ethics goes beyond the moral sense of right and wrong and is a systematic approach grounded in philosophical principles and theory. To apply ethical reasoning in clinical settings, it is necessary to be able to differentiate among ethics, morality, and the law.

Often healthcare professionals, including nurses, assume that *ethics* refers to how individuals feel morally, in other words, shared beliefs about right and wrong that influence how conduct occurs in a society. Although this may reflect concepts of common *morality*, *ethics* is more accurately defined as a practical discipline that provides rules or guidance for how one should act in consideration of others and not necessarily how one feels or believes (Pojman & Fieser, 2017). Given the complexity and diversity of the environments in which healthcare services are provided, it is important to appropriately apply ethical reasoning and refrain from making decisions solely on the basis of moral beliefs that may include value-laden judgments.

ETHICAL ISSUE, DISTRESS, OR DILEMMA

There is no replacement for careful deliberation regarding the ethical implications of an action. Often one is unaware of how to proceed when encountering an ethical issue, ethical distress, or ethical dilemma. The first step is to be able to differentiate among these varying situations. *Ethical issues* are conflicts that may occur frequently with many patients and are a concern for the profession as a whole. For example, ethical issues common to nursing practice may include noncompliance with a plan of treatment, parents who choose not to vaccinate their children, and complex end-of-life decisions.

Ethical distress relates to the painful feelings and psychological disequilibrium that result from a moral conflict in which one knows the correct action to take but constraints prevent implementation of the action (Jameton, 1984). It is often called *moral distress* because practitioners feel like they may have to compromise their values when providing or limiting treatment. Moral distress is prevalent in nursing practice and is linked to situations where nurses are asked to continue to provide treatment when the chance of recovery is poor. Nurses are often caught in the middle between physician providers and the patient's family, which also significantly contributes to feelings of moral distress.

An *ethical dilemma* occurs when one is confronted with two competing courses of action that appear to be morally obligatory. Ethical dilemmas also can occur when a nurse is required to make a decision and must act, but all courses of action violate an ethical principle, for example, when there is disagreement between family members about continued aggressive and burdensome interventions for an aged adult at the end of life.

RESOLUTION OF ETHICAL DILEMMAS

When encountering an ethical dilemma, nurses will often attempt to avoid conflict by collapsing ethical dilemmas into medical or legal questions. This capulizing allows them to defer decision making to those with expertise in the law or medicine. Again, although it is important to clarify clinical and legal implications to engage in diligent ethical analysis, ethical dilemmas should not be collapsed into medical or legal questions. Historically, the legal system has been ill-equipped to address complex medical decisions.

When ethical conflict arises, the values of the patient need to be balanced with what is medically indicated. Once decision making is deferred to the courts, legal counsel, or quality risk management, the patient's needs cease to be the focus of resolution. Instead, decisions are made in the best interest of the practitioners and/or organization. The ethical response can be realized only when those stakeholders who understand and can execute actions aimed at reasonable goals of care remain central to the shared decision-making process.

LAW VERSUS ETHICS

Although the *law* and *ethics* are similar, the legal course of action is not always ethically supported and vice versa. In other words, knowing what is legally permissible does not necessarily reveal what is ethical. Conversely, illegality is not akin to unethical conduct; however, many codes of ethics require healthcare professionals to comply with laws and regulations. Violating these standards means that the clinicians may risk losing their license or face other disciplinary action. Clinicians need to learn how to operate within the framework of the law. However, regardless of pressures associated when working in a litigious environment, every nurse has a personal and professional responsibility to provide ethically supported care.

EXPERTISE AND ETHICS

The other common mistake made by healthcare practitioners, including nurses, is to generalize expertise in the clinical healthcare arena to ethics. In the area of medicine, physicians often are assumed to have expertise in ethical aspects of decision making on the basis of their expertise about the technical facts (Fletcher, Lombardo, Marshall, & Miller, 1997). Thus, the mistake of defaulting to the physician's recommendation regarding ethical decisions is often made. It is important to recognize that all members of the treating team must be involved in the ethical-reasoning process. In cases in which conflict exists among members of the clinical team, nurse managers may have to step in to resolve it, as they may be able to communicate with physicians and other healthcare professionals in a way that minimizes power imbalances (Brandt, 2007).

In addition to the differentiation between ethics and morality, ethics and the law, and ethics and clinical expertise, ethicists commonly distinguish between approaches used in ethical deliberation.

APPROACHES TO ETHICAL ANALYSIS

Ethical theories relate to the study of right and wrong conduct in society, and in healthcare relate to how clinicians should behave. There are different approaches to defining ethics, but in healthcare, normative ethics guides standards of practice. A normative ethics approach is devoted to examining our moral relations with one another and guides nurses in how they should act in consideration of their patients. To determine the most ethical course of action, normative ethics asks questions about our fundamental duties, values, and virtues, what it means to be a role model, and whether the ends justify the means (Shafer-Landau, 2012). In clinical settings, when ethics committees and ethics consultants engage with healthcare teams to determine the best course of action for the patient, they are mainly doing normative ethics. Some may argue that nurses are engaged in what some consider a fourth kind of ethics, applied ethics. In medical or clinical contexts, *applied ethics* is the act of applying general moral theories and principles to ethical problems in practice (Brannigan & Boss, 2001). However, many consider applied ethics a type or subgroup of normative ethics, not a separate ethical approach; both normative and applied ethics focus on the practical task of determining the moral standards that should shape behavior.

Normative ethical approaches dominate ethics discussions in healthcare as they are linked to determining the rightness of an action. Although normative ethical approaches generally focus on either the act itself or the consequence of the action, there are multiple normative theories which may inform ethical decision making in practice. Understanding these theories and how they relate to practice may improve the ethical reasoning skills of practitioners and improve their ability to resolve and/or mitigate ethical conflicts in practice. Ethical theories are often criticized for their attempt to reduce everything down to that one viewpoint (Steinbock, London, & Arras, 2013). Theories provide a framework for addressing ethical quandaries in practice, but all theories if applied unilaterally may result in suboptimal outcomes; thus, although the philosophical arguments that ground these theories are not intended to be used together, in practice integrating differing approaches may better assist the practitioner in arriving at an ethically supported course of action (Brannigan & Boss, 2001). Various normative ethical theories, which may assist nurses to effectively analyze complex ethical problems, are described in the following text.

Normative Ethical Theories

Even though clinical ethics can be categorized as an imprecise discipline, the following ethical theories are predicated on the assumption that there are objective moral truths. Although each theory subscribes to a different approach in defining moral truth or ethically supported action, the theories presume that ethics is neither relative nor subjective and that there is such a thing as morality, and conversely immoral action. Even though there are many complex questions in clinical ethics, which may make it difficult to define an objective good, the ethical course of action is one that is supported by reason. An act is judged to be ethical if it is backed by better reasons than alternatives (Rachels & Rachels, 2015). In clinical ethics, the objective claims, or moral truths, regarding right and wrong conduct are generally linked to one of the following four families of theories: Virtue Ethics, Ethics of Care, Consequentialism, and Deontology.

Virtue Ethics

The theory of virtue ethics focuses less on the moral action and instead is concerned with the character of the moral agent (the person who is completing the action). Contemporary virtue ethics can be traced back to the philosophy of the ancient Greeks and, specifically, Aristotle's *Nicomachean Ethics* (Steinbock et al., 2013). According to one of the themes of Virtue Ethics, a right action is understood in reference to what a virtuous person would do (Shafer-Landau, 2012). Opposition to this theory stems from the subjective nature of defining ethical action on the seemingly arbitrary nature of why and how a "virtuous" person may choose to act. However, in the complex world of healthcare, many would argue that a theory where the nuances of ethical decision making can be addressed is preferred. Proponents of virtue theory argue that, secondary to the complexity of most ethical problems, the right action "cannot be adequately captured by a set of rules" and therefore the moral agent must also rely on one's virtue that has been cultivated in experience (Steinbock et al., 2013, p. 33). The virtuous person would be able to use reason to support the action taken on the basis of the facts of the situation, morally relevant variables, emotional maturity, and application of past experience. The following vignette provides an account of a virtuous practitioner.

VIGNETTE 4.1: VIRTUE ETHICS

Veronica is a nurse who has been practicing for over 25 years. Over the course of the past 15 years, she has been working in a clinic where she is a valued mentor to her colleagues and has an impeccable reputation as a thoughtful, compassionate, and honest practitioner. During annual peer reviews, her colleagues consistently praise her for "going above and beyond" when caring for her patients. When Veronica's colleagues encounter ethical dilemmas, they often go to her for advice. Veronica has shown great insight when identifying which ethical principles are in conflict, applying her past experience to weigh possible consequences, and then making a reasoned decision regarding the best course of action.

Her colleagues believe her to exhibit integrity and strong character. Therefore, they trust that she will provide them with sound advice when faced with making ethical decisions.

Ethics of Care

Ethics requires us to make decisions in consideration of others, so it can be subsumed that ethics by nature is relational. "Whether concerned with justice, character, motivation, right action or living well, ethics evaluates the implications of one's agency on others and their agency on one's self. This concept is embraced by the ethics of care" (Corcoran, Brandt, Fleming, & Gu, 2016, p. 3). Ethics of Care is a relationship-based theory, meaning that it focuses on compassion and empathy rather than on the character of the moral agent. This ethical theory can be traced back to the work of Carol Gilligan, who objected to the notion that an ethic of principles is a higher order of moral development than an ethic on the basis of relationships (Gilligan, 1982). This theory continues to be closely identified with modern feminist philosophy, as women typically respond in terms of relational caring, whereas men typically reason in terms of duty and justice (Rachels & Rachels, 2015). Ethics of care is reflective of virtue ethics in that it is not focused on the action itself, but rather how the moral agent executes the action. However, it deviates from virtue ethics in that it is less focused on the character of the moral agent and more on promotion of a caring relationship.

Although the ethics of care holds promise as a viable theory, especially in nursing that is predicated on a caring relationship, there are many pitfalls associated with this theory when not tempered with an objective moral norm. Specifically, the ethics of care theory has been criticized for the following limitations: threatening to restrict the scope of the moral community, emotions related to caring relationships clouding judgment, lack of impartiality, lack of strategy in dealing with uncooperative/dangerous people, and a lack of accommodation for moral rights (Shafer-Landau, 2012). Although the ethics of care has substantial value in nursing practice as it promotes a caring empathetic response to client needs, the following vignette outlines the limitations of the theory when not used in concert with accepted moral standards or principles.

VIGNETTE 4.2: ETHICS OF CARE

David is a nurse who works in a public health clinic. One of the primary barriers for his patients is that they are unable to afford reliable transportation to attend regular clinic visits. David has a friend who works for the transit system. He tells David that he has access to free public transit passes, which he has permission to distribute to disgruntled passengers who threaten to file a complaint. He offers to give David a stack of passes to disseminate to patients, stating, "Even though your patients don't technically meet the criteria for a free pass, it doesn't really hurt anything." According to the ethics of care theory, David would work with his friend to distribute the free passes to patients who he believes would most benefit. His focus is on the patient relationship, not impartial rules. Nonetheless, deliberate misuse of public resources is clearly unethical.

Consequentialism

Consequentialism, also referred to as teleological theory, derives ethical merit by focusing on the outcome of an action. One of the most recognized consequentialist theories is utilitarianism. *Utility*, or the overall usefulness of an action, is described as doing the greatest good for the greatest number of people. Ultimately the morally right action is the action that has the best effect, either maximizing good or limiting harm. Consequentialism typically involves asking the following questions (Pozgar, 2012, p. 7):

What will be the effects of each course of action?

Will they be positive or negative?

Who will benefit?

What will do the least harm?

Consequentialism is criticized most often for its innate incompatibility with justice, especially with regard to the potential impact on the minority as well as its focus on backward-looking reasoning (Rachels & Rachels, 2015). This theory is concerned with the utility argument, so to attain the greatest good for the greatest number, it supports committing an injustice that impacts only the minority of individuals as long as the action produces benefit for the majority. In addition, consequentialism predicates its ethical rationale on the outcome of an action that has yet to take place. One of the strongest defenses of these criticisms is that the principle of utility should be used as a guide for choosing rules (i.e., rule utilitarianism), not as a guide for supporting individual acts (i.e., act utilitarianism).

VIGNETTE 4.3: ACT VERSUS RULE UTILITARIAN

Bobby is a charge nurse in the medical intensive care unit (ICU), and all beds are full. Mr. Jones is a 78-year-old patient in the ICU who is in intubated status after an acute stroke that left him unable to communicate with his family or care team. Neurology has been consulted and feels that his long-term neurologic prognosis is poor. The team all agrees that it would be clinically appropriate to transition the patient to palliative care and out of the ICU; however, the patient's family wants to "do everything, in order to see him fight to live another day." The ventilatory support is not biomedically futile, but the team feels that, given the patient's poor prognosis, continued ventilatory support is not ethically or clinically indicated. The ICU has begun diverting patients to other hospitals as there are no beds, and Bobby is getting pressure from the nurses and physicians to have Mr. Jones transferred to the floor to admit more ICU-"appropriate" patients.

Deontology

Rule utilitarianism may seem to resolve some of the ethical critiques associated with a consequential approach; however, this begs the question of how to establish the moral worth of certain rules. In the case given earlier, is the limited effectiveness or benefit of the action more ethically persuasive or is respecting the patient's autonomy by allowing the family to determine goals of care as long as procedures are not clearly biomedically futile a higher ethical priority? Complicating the case further is the concept of access to care or justice.

Deontology is a rule-based or duty-based theory. In contrast to consequentialism, deontology focuses on the action as opposed to the consequence of that action. The Ten Commandments and the Golden Rule are common examples of deontology. The primary philosophical critique of religion-based rules or treating others as one would want to be treated is that the rules themselves are not universal. One of the most recognized and important philosophers to refute utilitarianism and propose the idea of using universal norms to determine ethical action was Immanuel Kant.

Kant believed that persons cannot be used as a means to an ends, and focused his work on demonstrating through reason that there are categorical imperatives that must be universally adopted. According to Kant's categorical imperative, one should "act only according to that maxim whereby you can at the same time will that it should become a universal law" (Ellington, 1993, p. 30). By this standard, the golden rule falls short in healthcare settings; the idea that we should treat our clients as we want to be treated may in some cases require us to provide interventions not valued by our clients. Even though there is reasonable concern with using the Golden Rule to guide decision making in healthcare, ethicists such as Beauchamp and Childress argue that there are universally accepted rules which should be used to guide healthcare decisions. These rules are known as the Principles of Biomedical Ethics. Although this principles-based approach (principlism) differs from

Kant's universal law theory, in the rules themselves as well as the concept of absolute duty, it still subscribes to a deontological normative theory.

Arguably the most commonly used framework in contemporary Western healthcare ethics is principlism as outlined by Beauchamp and Childress (Brannigan & Boss, 2001). In 1979, Beauchamp and Childress published *Principles of Biomedical Ethics*, which was predicated on the four principles outlined in the Belmont Report. The authors contended that the four principles of beneficence, nonmaleficence, justice, and respect for autonomy are useful in guiding ethical decision making in healthcare. According to principlism, when consequences and principles conflict, the ethical act is the one in accordance with the principles. The principles are not like universal laws; as Beauchamp and Childress state, "It is a mistake in biomedical ethics to assign priority to any basic principle over other basic principles—as if morality must be hierarchically structured or as if we must cherish one moral norm over another without consideration of particular circumstances" (2013, p. ix).

VIGNETTE 4.4: PRINCIPLISM

Jamal is a home healthcare nurse. His patient is a 90-year-old male, who suffered from a stroke and now cannot move independently or feed himself. In addition, the patient is nearly 6 feet 2 inches tall and weighs 220 pounds. He insisted on going home from rehabilitation, stating his family will take care of him. The discharging healthcare team had concerns about discharge home because his wife is 89 years old and significantly smaller than her husband; in addition, she has sustained recent compression fractures to the spine. Rehabilitation agreed to the discharge plan because the daughter said she would help. Within a week, it becomes apparent that the daughter is unable to assist, and 911 has been called three times this week to assist with getting him up after he has fallen as his wife is unable to manage him. The patient continues to insist that he has a right to be home, even though his wife is now pleading with him to go to the nursing home for additional rehabilitation and potentially to stay as she is feeling overwhelmed. He refuses to leave the home and Jamal, respecting the patient's autonomy, convinces the wife that he should remain at home.

Practical Strategies to Promote Ethical Practice

Advanced practice nurses, including nurse practitioners, clinical nurse specialists, nurse-midwives, and certified nurse anesthetists, will inevitably encounter situations that pose ethical challenges. These may relate to the interaction between the practitioner and the client, relationships and actions between colleagues, and the impact of administrative directives, which may override clinical judgment in the current, reimbursement-driven healthcare environment. This chapter focuses on providing resources to develop and enhance ethical reasoning in practitioners with a goal of increased ability to identify, analyze, and ultimately resolve ethical dilemmas.

Ethical situations can be complex and the best course of action to resolve them can be ambiguous. A systematic, step-by-step method of analysis, including incorporating strategies for ethical decision making such as those outlined in Box 4.1, can help the practitioner to arrive at a plan of action that best resolves or manages the dilemma. These dilemmas can be complicated, so practitioners are advised to use all available ethics resources, including the nursing Code of Ethics and, where available, ethics committees.

There are many strategies, frameworks, and processes developed to strategically address ethical dilemmas in practice; however, the core elements are similar. They are designed to identify all potential players who may be affected by the decision, as well as gather information from broad sources to ensure that the eventual decision considers all aspects of the situation and potential actions with likely outcomes of each. It is also useful to consider the potential unintended consequences of the decision. Practitioners should be aware that not making a decision, hoping someone else will deal with the issue, is also a decision but the situation may continue to be problematic and troubling. Ethical dilemmas are challenging and require a systematic method of analysis to ensure that all relevant information is obtained and all potential actions (and their likely results) are considered to arrive at a decision that can be defended.

BOX 4.1 Strategies for Ethical Decision Making

Ensure that involved parties have their voices heard.
Ethical dilemmas should not be collapsed into legal questions.
Clinical reasoning must accompany ethical analysis.
Expertise in the clinical healthcare arena should not be generalized to ethics.
Disclose and be aware of own moral values and bias.

Source: Adapted from Fletcher, J. C., Lombardo, P. A., Marshall, M. F., & Miller, F. G. (Eds.) (1997). *Introduction to Clinical Ethics* (2nd ed.). Hagerstown, MD: University Publishing Group.

CRITICAL THINKING QUESTIONS

1. Share an ethical dilemma you have experienced as a nurse. How was the problem solved? Could it have been handled in a better way?

2. How does the process of resolving ethical dilemmas relate to general problem solving?

3. Provide a clinical example of an ethical dilemma, ethical issue, or ethical distress and identify which one it is. What makes it a dilemma, issue, or distress?

4. Create a clinical scenario where ethics would conflict with the law. Then, discuss how you would work through the issue.

REFERENCES

Beauchamp, T. L., & Childress, J. F. (2013). *Principles of biomedical ethics* (7th ed.). New York, NY: Oxford University Press.

Brandt, L. (2007). Organizational ethics. *OT Practice, 12*(21)15–19.

Brannigan, M. C., & Boss, J. A. (2001). *Healthcare ethics in a diverse society.* Mountain View, CA: Mayfield.

Corcoran, B. C., Brandt, L., Fleming, D. A., & Gu, C. N. (2016). Fidelity to the healing relationship: A medical student's challenge to contemporary bioethics and prescription for medical practice. *Journal of Medical Ethics, 42*(4), 224–228. doi:10.1136/medethics-2013-101718

Ellington, J. W. (1993). *Immanuel Kant: Grounding for the metaphysics of morals; On a supposed right to lie because of philanthropic concerns* (3rd ed.). Indianapolis/ Cambridge, IN: Hackett Publishing.

Fletcher, J. C., Lombardo, P. A., Marshall, M. F., & Miller, F. G. (Eds.) (1997). *Introduction to Clinical Ethics* (2nd ed.). Hagerstown, MD: University Publishing Group.

Gilligan, C. (1982). *In a different voice.* Cambridge, MA: Harvard University Press.

Jameton, A. (1984). *Nursing Practice: The Ethical Issues.* Englewood Cliffs, NJ: Prentice Hall.

Pojman, L. P., & Fieser, J. (2017). *Ethics: Discovering right and wrong* (8th ed.). Belmont, CA: Thomson Wadsworth.

Pozgar, G. D. (2012). *Legal and ethical issues for health professionals* (3rd ed.). Burlington, MA: Jones & Bartlett Learning.

Rachels, J., & Rachels, S. (2015). *The elements of moral philosophy* (8th ed.). Boston, MA: McGraw-Hill.

Shafer-Landau, R. (2012). *The fundamentals of ethics* (2nd ed.). New York, NY: Oxford University Press.

Steinbock, B., London, A. J., & Arras, J. (2013). *Ethical issues in modern medicine: Contemporary readings in bioethics* (8th ed.). New York, NY: McGraw-Hill.

SECTION II

MSN Roles

Sections II and III are divided by direct and indirect care roles of master's-prepared nurses. The roles for this book were chosen from the list provided by the American Association of Colleges of Nursing (AACN) given in Chapter 2. One very important notation to make is that the roles discussed in this book are in no way all-inclusive. One of the beautiful traits of the nursing profession is the plethora of different things to do and learn coupled with the ever-changing landscape. In this section, we take a look at the clinical nurse leader, educator, and advanced practice care roles. Again, with the wide range of opportunities in the advanced practice care realm, this book takes a topical look at all of these roles. However, discussion of each role provides an understanding of the history of the role and information to give you an idea of what that particular role is all about.

CHAPTER 5

MSN as Clinical Nurse Leader

Amanda S. Brown

OBJECTIVES

1. Explain how the clinical nurse leader (CNL) role developed.
2. Examine theories used as a CNL.
3. Describe ethical issues that the CNL needs to be aware of.
4. Apply ethics to the CNL role.

The CNL role is the first new nursing role in over 30 years. The Institute of Medicine (IOM) brought attention to critical healthcare concerns in 1999 that triggered the American Association of Colleges of Nursing (AACN) to address safety and quality gaps in care.

HISTORY OF THE ROLE

In 1999, the IOM published a report, *To Err Is Human*, suggesting that healthcare was not as safe as it should be and that between 44,000 and 98,000 people in hospitals died annually because of medical errors related to hospitals' lack of systems, processes, and poor conditions (IOM, 1999). A second report was published in 2001, *Chasing the Quality Chasm: A New Health System for the 21st Century*, putting the focus on the aging population and the need to address the treatment of chronic conditions over acute episodic care (IOM, 2001). The report also noted that the healthcare delivery system is poorly organized and too complex to meet the needs of the challenges at hand. Six specific aims for quality improvement were identified: Patient care should be safe, effective, patient-centered, timely, efficient, and equitable (IOM, 2001). To help achieve the six aims, the *Quality Chasm* report identifies 10 rules for health system redesign:

1. Care is based on continuous healing relationships.

2. Care is customized according to patient needs and values.

3. The patient is the source of control.

4. Knowledge is shared and information flows freely.

5. Decision making is evidence based.

6. Safety is a system property.

7. Transparency is necessary.

8. Needs are anticipated.

9. Waste is continuously decreased.

10. Cooperation among clinicians is a priority.

Along with the need to improve patient care outcomes, there was also talk of a national nursing shortage in the early 2000s. There was an increased demand for registered nursing (RN) services because of high levels of retirement and the increased aging population and low enrollment in education programs, predicting that the United States would be short 1 million nurses by 2020 (Clarke, 2016).

The AACN began working on a solution to address the challenges faced by the healthcare systems. In 2003, the AACN unveiled the initial white paper outlining the expectations of a new role in nursing, the CNL, which would address healthcare outcome concerns, the needs of the aging population, and the nursing profession (Sotomayor & Rankin, 2017).

EDUCATION AND CERTIFICATION

The CNL is an advanced clinician with a master of science in nursing (MSN) degree and specialty CNL certification. Graduate education is necessary because the CNL is the expert at the point of care and must have a higher level of clinical competence and knowledge to serve as a resource (AACN, 2004). There are currently three AACN board-approved educational models. Models were developed to accommodate bachelor of science in nursing (BSN) program graduates, associate degree in nursing (ADN) graduates (RN to MSN), and MSN graduates with a post-master's certificate (AACN, 2017a).

The AACN collaborated with practice partners, public consumers, and a professional test development agency to develop a certification examination to credential individuals who have graduated or are preparing to graduate from the CNL MSN degree programs. Individuals who are eligible to sit for the CNL certification exam are those who have graduated from the CNL MSN program and completed all practice hours, as well as individuals in the final term of their CNL education who meet the criteria described by the CNL Curriculum Framework identified in the AACN's Competency and Curricular Expectations for the Clinical Nurse Leader Education and Practice (AACN, 2017a). Those who have passed the CNL certification exam and have a license to practice as an RN earn the CNL credential (AACN, 2017a).

CLINICAL NURSE LEADER ROLE AND COMPETENCIES

The CNL is trained to work across the continuum of care within any healthcare setting. It is not a management role or administrative, and implementation can vary across different settings (AACN, 2017b). The CNL is positioned at the frontline of care, ensuring other healthcare workers within the multidisciplinary team are engaged in providing their own clinical care (Bender, 2017), and collaborates with the unit manager to assist in the function of the unit. The CNL role includes working as a healthcare provider at the microsystem, or unit, level for day-to-day activities; performing comprehensive health assessments of patients, family, and caregivers; initiating, continuing, and adjusting patient care plans; and assuming accountability and responsibility for education, care delivery, and outcomes within the microsystem for patients, families, and nurses (Baker, Rushing, True, & Rodriguez, 2015). There are several different variations, but the core competencies of the CNL role include lateral integration of care through interdisciplinary teams, member and leader of healthcare teams, skillful communication within the multidisciplinary teams, and implementation of an interdisciplinary approach to safe, quality patient care (Moore, Schmidt, & Howington, 2014, p. 190).

So, what exactly does a CNL do every day? For starters, a CNL is not expected to take a staff nurse–patient assignment (Duffey, 2017), cover for staff nurse breaks, or fill in when units are short staffed. CNLs are responsible for rounding on their patients daily, and during rounds, the CNL reviews the patient's medical records, ensuring the correct protocols are being followed on the basis of the individual diagnosis and clinical status (Sheets et al., 2012). Part of the CNL role is prevention; during rounds, the CNL will assess all designated patients for any risk factors, such as falls, skin breakdown, and deep vein thrombosis (DVT). Assessment of invasive devices, dates of insertion, and appropriateness of the devices, such as chest tubes, indwelling urinary catheters, and central venous catheters, is part of rounding, as well as ensuring removal of the devices when no longer necessary. The CNL also assesses for any support service needs, such as dietary, physical therapy, and occupational therapy. The CNL communicates with the interdisciplinary team and makes referrals for patient appointments. Communication with the interdisciplinary team is a crucial part of the CNL role when needs are identified; the CNL works closely with the patient care team. For example, if a patient is diagnosed with a hospital-acquired pressure ulcer, the CNL contacts the wound/ostomy care team for an assessment. Once the wound/ostomy care team assesses the patient and places wound care orders, the CNL re-educates the staff nurses on proper turning, repositioning, and strategies for reducing skin breakdown and pressure ulcers. The CNL then monitors the ulcer daily along with staff compliance and communication to ensure a positive outcome. If necessary, one-on-one training is provided to staff nurses. The CNL should meet daily with the multidisciplinary team to discuss discharge and discharge needs; the CNL reports on all patients and works with the team to reduce the average length of stay (LOS), ensuring patients are ready for discharge to reduce readmission rates. CNLs are available to assist staff nurses with bedside procedures, for example, if an order is placed for an indwelling urinary catheter and the staff nurse is unsure about the proper procedure, the CNL can walk the staff nurse through the procedure and offer support. Along with responsibilities on the unit, the CNL belongs to several different hospital committees, such as the wound/ostomy care committee, and remains current on evidence-based practices. CNLs monitor for trends and assess for areas of improvement on the unit and use evidence-based practice to update policies and procedures. The CNL then develops a process improvement plan and implements a change of practice on the unit. The following is a case study reviewing how a CNL implements change within the microsystem.

VIGNETTE 5.1

A 27-bed medical–surgical unit had over 90 falls in 1 year. The CNL assessed the postfall debriefings, looked at trends, and found that the majority were falling while attempting to ambulate to the bathroom; the facility had recently rid the units of the ability to use waist restraints on patients who were high fall risks. After completing a literature review, the CNL learned communication enhancements that led to positive outcomes and developed a plan. The CNL updated the Kardex to address fall risk assessment, preventative measures, and interventions if a bed/chair alarm was needed and fall history. The CNL trained the staff nurses on bed alarms and chair alarms to ensure proper use of both. Whiteboards in the patient rooms were also updated with ambulation method and any necessary devices. A calendar was placed in the break room and the number of falls was captured along with the time of day for each day a fall occurred. The calendar was used to remind the nurses of the goal to reduce the fall rate and as a reminder to communicate ambulation methods at bedside report. Daily rounds by the CNL were necessary to ensure the staff was compliant with the practice changes; if nurses were not communicating, re-education was provided. The CNL with the collaboration of the microsystem was able to reduce the fall rate by over 50% in 1 year.

THEORY RELATED TO THE CNL ROLE

A theory commonly associated with the CNL role is the transition theory (TT). The TT is a middle range theory conceived by Afaf Ibrahim Meleis while working through her master's and PhD dissertation (Im, 2014). The purpose of the theory was to better understand, explain, and describe the different experiences of human beings in a variety of transitions (Im, 2014). Transition is a result frequently experienced in life through health; nurses are often the primary contact for patients and families while undergoing transition during medical treatment (Meleis, Sawyer, Im, Hilfinger Messias, & Schumacher, 2000). Nurses at the point of care are the ones who prepare patients for impending transitions and facilitate the process of learning new skills related to the patients' health and illness experiences (Meleis et al., 2000). The CNL works within the microsystem to improve communication and make transitions smooth for patients and families. Examples of transitions experienced by patients and families that can make them vulnerable are illness experiences, diagnosis, surgical procedures, rehabilitation, and recovery; developmental life-span transitions, adolescence, menopause, aging, pregnancy, parenthood, adolescence, and death; and social and cultural transitions such as retirement and members taking on the role of caregiver (Meleis et al., 2000). The TT provides a fitting framework with which CNLs will be able to assist patients, families, and nurses during times of constant changes in their health and illness.

Given the increase in the number of ethnically diverse patient populations in the United States, the CNL needs to be aware of and culturally sensitive to these patients who are experiencing transition and have different perspectives on health and illness (Maag, Buccheri, Capella, & Jennings, 2006).

The TT suggests that three factors, individual, community, and social, all regarding culture, education, and social status, can influence the patients' type, patterns, and properties of transitions (Meleis et al., 2000). The theory provides the CNL with the culturally sensitive knowledge that will assist the CNL in working with ethnically diverse patients during times of transition from a state of illness to that of optimal health.

ETHICAL CONSIDERATIONS

The CNL is responsible for overseeing, facilitating, and coordinating care across the microsystem. As a leader, the CNL must provide ethical leadership. Ethical leadership means the CNL must make professional ethical decisions and lead ethically in everyday practice, in all interactions, and in health promotion of the organization by respecting moral concepts and the law, while also respecting the different beliefs and values of others. The best way for the CNL to promote quality care is by integrating health policy, ethics, and advocacy into all nursing interventions (Harris & Roussel, 2010). The CNL works as the spokesperson and is in a position to collaborate with resources, such as the ethics committee, to resolve ethical matters. Furthermore, the CNL has the ability to see the big picture, be the voice, and take part in solving the big picture issue. The following case study provides examples of how the CNL assists with microsystem ethical considerations.

VIGNETTE 5.2

During morning rounds on a medical–surgical unit, a surgical resident requests supplies to insert a chest tube. The staff nurse caring for the patient is a newly graduated nurse and is not comfortable with the process of bedside chest tube placement. The staff nurse asks the CNL for assistance. As the CNL is showing the staff nurse where to find the bedside procedure checklist and paperwork, the surgeon becomes impatient and begins to gather his own supplies. The CNL reminds the surgeon that the staff nurse will need to look up his credentials and ensure he is trained and certificated to insert the chest tube without the supervision of his chief. The surgeon says he is able and going to do it; the CNL could see the staff nurse hesitation in continuing to follow the policy and encourages her to continue looking up the information and completing all necessary documentation. The staff nurse verifies that the surgeon is trained and clear to continue, paperwork is completed, and the disgruntled surgeon begins to insert the chest tube. After the patient is prepped and the surgeon grabs the chest tube, it slips out of his hand and lands on the floor; the surgeon picks the tube up and prepares to insert it into the patient. The staff nurse looked at the CNL concerned but hesitant to say anything; as the surgeon went to reinsert the dirty chest tube, the CNL stepped in and stopped the surgeon from inserting the tube. The CNL was able to step out of the room and obtain new supplies and the tube was inserted with no additional complications.

The staff nurse and the CNL debriefed after the procedure and discussed the situation. The CNL talks with the new staff nurse about difficult situations where it is necessary to speak up and advocate for the patient. The staff nurse mentioned that the surgeon and his aggression intimidated her. This made her fearful to say anything and that is why she waited on the CNL to step in. The CNL assured the staff nurse that she will always be supported when speaking up for what is in the best interest of the patient and encouraged her to always use her voice. The CNL then scheduled a meeting with the unit manager, surgeon, and chief of surgery to discuss the main concerns of patient safety, policy and procedure compliance, and the role of the staff nurse to advocate for the patient.

IMPLEMENTATION OF THE ROLE

A key element of the CNL role is to establish a relationship between education and practice to produce empowerment, quality enhancement, shared resources, and integrated services, and to improve outcomes (Moore et al., 2014). The CNL role has been identified as an innovative new role to improve care environments, patient safety, and quality outcomes (Bender, 2016), and to be a catalyst for change. However, for the role to have a positive impact on the unit, the introduction and implementation of the role are important. The introduction and implementation of the role can be difficult because the standardization of the role varies.

The first step is for leadership to define the role, ensuring that the interprofessional team fully understands how the role functions on a day-to-day basis within the microsystem (Duffey, 2017). If the CNL role is not clearly understood and the CNL is used to cover breaks, complete administrative duties, or take a patient assignment when the staff nurse numbers are down, outcomes may not change for the unit. Preparing the staff and those at the bedside is crucial for a collaborative success; studies have shown significant problems with implementation when all members of the team do not show support prior to the implementation (Duffey, 2017). The staff should be educated on the role expectations. Duffey (2017) suggested the use of implementation teams, pilot studies prior to full implementation, educating the staff on how the CNL interacts with the team, role duties, and the influence the role has on positive patient outcomes. Stakeholder involvement, standardization, and education about the CNL role are crucial for implementation and the success of the CNL.

INTERVIEW

The following interview was conducted with a CNL currently working on a medical, surgical, and telemetry unit that houses 22 patients. Positive aspects, as well as struggles encountered while working on the unit, are discussed.

Author: How long have you been in the CNL role?

CNL: I started to function in the role of CNL in February 2017.

Author: What is a typical day like for a CNL?

CNL: This has been a huge discussion and topic for many CNLs I have reached out to. CNLs are able to function on any unit, in any healthcare setting; therefore, a typical day and a normal routine do not really exist. I reached out to many CNLs when I first started with the flat-out question, "What am I supposed to do?" As this seems so elementary to ask fellow colleagues, I was bombarded with responses as others were plagued with the same questions. For myself, I start my day with doing a walkthrough of the unit and check on the patients as to any issues that occurred overnight that need to be addressed and discuss them with their medical teams. I then participate in discharge planning, which includes a multidisciplinary team that discusses each patient on each unit and what his or her specific needs for discharge may be, how his or her treatment is progressing, and so forth. This provides me with the opportunity to get a picture of not only the patients on my unit but the patients on other units as well. This also gives me an understanding of what discharges to expect for that day or what patients had any "cardiac events" overnight and may need telemetry monitoring. After the discharge meeting, I relay all the pertinent information to the bedside nurses, so they have an idea of what to expect for that patient that day. With the patients mentioned in discharge planning, I am able to focus on individual ones with their primary concerns, whether it is additional education on diabetes, warfarin teaching, Foley catheter care, and so forth. Many items that the bedside nurses might not have time to complete. I am involved in many committees where at least one typically occurs every day; Wednesdays are meeting days and they really seem back to back. I am involved with staff competencies and maintaining our up-to-date status. There is monthly competency and it usually takes a month to get the whole unit signed off. Lastly, I have made my schedule where I continue to, on 2 days, have a patient assignment. I wanted it to be known that I was different from management and administration and still considered an equal with my fellow staff nurses despite my advanced degree.

Author: Do you cover nursing shortages on your unit? If so, how often and does this affect your ability to meet the role expectations?

CNL: Nursing shortages happen quite frequently as they do in any hospital setting. On days that I am slotted to function as the CNL and I get pulled, then yes, this does affect the ability to meet my role expectations. Although, as mentioned in the previous question, I still do have some days that are designated as floor staff days; that is my choice.

Author: Do you feel like you are able to function fully in your role?

CNL: I do not feel as though I am able to fully function in my role. It has been extremely difficult to gain acceptance with not only floor staff but upper management as well. My immediate managers have been wonderful, as I have been working with them the entire time I was in school. Because this is a new role, it has been a difficult transition and informing additional staff of what exactly I am supposed to be doing. A lot of time and effort has gone into providing upper management with the "white paper" and proving with an evidence-based practice that the CNL will provide great advancements if utilized correctly on each unit.

Author: Do you feel other nurses fully understand your role? If not, what do you wish they could understand?

CNL: One hundred percent of other nurses do not fully understand my role. They believe I am part of the administration and upper management and do not understand I have no additional power than they do. I have met and continue to meet great resistance with any attempts to implement new ideas or skills onto the unit. I do believe this will get better as my role becomes more clearly defined.

Author: Do you feel that the multidisciplinary team within your facility fully understands your role? If not, what do you wish they could better understand?

CNL: I do not believe the multidisciplinary team understands my role and exactly how to utilize the skills I have that can greatly affect patient needs and care. I have introduced myself to many ancillary staff members as the Clinical Nurse Leader and the same individuals will refer to me as the Nurse

Educator. Although the role has been around for only a couple years, it still is quite unfamiliar to many. More representation of what the Clinical Nurse Leader has to offer and the specific items I am able to assist with would be monumental.

Author: What type of unit do you work on? How many CNLs are in your facility? Do you work altogether? If so, what are some of your recent projects?

CNL: I currently am on a medical–surgical/telemetry unit. We house 22 inpatients with the capacity for 22 telemetry monitors along with ventilator patients and dialysis patients. There is one additional CNL in my facility; he works in the ICU. We are involved in many meetings and committees together and, when possible, we work together. The good thing is we went through schooling together, so we have created a bond. Together we have dealt with the ups and downs of introducing a new role into the hospital. Some of the recent projects I have been working on include:

a.   Created a binder as a quick reference for policies/procedures that pertain and are quite frequent on the unit.

b.   We previously had a welcome folder that was presented to all new admissions with information pertaining to the facility, our specific unit, and a place to write questions. These folders were looked at as another piece of paper, thrown out or left in the rooms by the patients after discharge. I am currently working on a binder with laminated copies that are able to remain in the patient room and cleaned on discharge, with information pertaining to the facility, the patient's stay, and any additional questions that the patient may think about and write down.

c.   Education plays a huge role throughout every admission. I am currently working with the discharge case manager and the diabetic educator on an easy-to-read-and-understand brochure for diabetic education postdischarge.

Author: What is the greatest accomplishment so far as the CNL?

CNL: I am proud of the policy and procedure binder I created. Staff have made multiple comments about how frequently the book is utilized and the amount of time it has saved. It was quite time-consuming to create, and I needed to research best practices for many things that were not in our current policies. The time and effort put forth have proven beneficial on so many fronts.

Author: What are the difficult aspects of the CNL role? What are the positive aspects?

CNL: I really think there have been more difficult aspects of the role than not. It has remained quite frustrating not getting the immediate staff buy-in and the multiple resistances we are met with on a daily basis. We are creating our own path, which is exciting but also unsettling. After reaching out to other CNLs, they have all said there is light at the end of the tunnel. All have met with some resistance or uncertainty, but all have ensured us it will get better.

Author: Is there anything else you think would be important for individuals learning about the CNL role to know?

CNL: I think it is important to understand how your facility views the Clinical Nurse Leader and what to expect. It is important that while you are going to school and if you are going to work in the facility you currently work in to start early and work with your nursing educators, human resources, managers, and staff to fully understand the role. I have become part of a mentor program, which has helped tremendously. My mentor has been a CNL for 6 years now and is my go-to person almost daily. She is currently in Minnesota, so we email back and forth. It gives me hope that she mentioned it took her a good 2 years to become established in her facility and have set tasks that are performed daily. This, again, makes me hopeful.

Before implementing the CNL role, the facility must have a vision for the role, manageable workload expectations, buy-in from all stakeholders, and a clear understanding of the role. Facilities that have less resistance to the role are those with organizational needs, desire to improve patient care and outcomes, opportunity to redesign care delivery, and desire to promote RN professional development and enhance physician–nurse relationships (King & Gerard, 2016).

SUMMARY

The CNL role can provide a great deal of opportunity for a unit to not only improve patient outcomes and reduce costs but also develop new nurses and provide an environment for innovation. Careful planning must go into the implementation and all stakeholders must be supportive in the process and offer continued support throughout implementation. The CNL has the knowledge and tools to respond to the demand to improve the quality of healthcare; it is the support within the macro- and microsystems that can ultimately influence the role and its desired outcomes.

CRITICAL THINKING QUESTIONS

1. Discuss your thoughts on the *Quality Chasm*. Is it good? Is it helpful? How will it guide your practice?

2. In considering the history of the CNL role, where do you see it going in the future?

3. Review the interview with the CNL. What responses surprise you and/or concern you?

4. Discuss your vision for how you would lead others in the CNL role.

REFERENCES

American Association of Colleges of Nursing. (2004). Talking points. Retrieved from http://www.aacnnursing.org/CNL/About/Talking-Points

American Association of Colleges of Nursing. (2017a). CNL frequently asked questions. Retrieved from http://www.aacnnursing.org/CNL/About/FAQs

American Association of Colleges of Nursing. (2017b). Competencies and curricular expectations for clinical nurse leader education and practice. Retrieved from http://www.aacnnursing.org/News-Information/Position-Statements-White-Papers/CNL

Baker, K. A., Rushing, J., True, B., & Rodriguez, L. (2015). A collaborative model for the CNL and CNS. *Nursing Management, 46*(7), 11–14. doi:10.1097/01.NUMA.0000466494.38698.13

Bender, M. (2016). Clinical nurse leader integration into practice: Developing theory to guide best practice. *Journal of Professional Nursing, 32*(1), 32–40. doi:10.1016/j.profnurs.2015.06.007

Bender, M. (2017). Clinical nurse leader-integrated care delivery: An approach to organizing nursing knowledge into practice models that promote interprofessional, team-based care. *Journal of Nursing Care Quality, 32*(3), 189–195. doi:10.1097/NCQ.0000000000000247

Clarke, S. P. (2016). RN workforce update: Current and long-range forecast. *Nursing Management, 47*(11), 20–25. doi:10.1097/01.NUMA.0000502798.99305.10

Duffey, P. (2017). Implementing the clinical nurse leader role in a large hospital network. *Nurse Leader, 15*(4), 276–280. doi:10.1016/j.mnl.2017.03.014

Harris, J. L., & Roussel, L. (2010). *Initiating and sustaining the clinical nurse leader role.* Sudbury, MA: Jones & Bartlett.

Im, E. O. (2014). Situation-specific theories from the middle-range transitions theory. *Advances in Nursing Science, 37*(1), 19–31. doi:10.1097/ANS.0000000000000014

Institute of Medicine. (1999). *To err is human: Building a safer health system*. Washington, DC: National Academies Press. Retrieved from http://www.nationalacademies.org/hmd/~/media/Files/Report%20Files/1999/To-Err-is-Human/To%20Err%20is%20Human%201999%20%20report%20brief.pdf

Institute of Medicine. (2001). *Crossing the quality chasm: A new health system for the 21st century*. Washington, DC: National Academies Press. Retrieved from http://www.nationalacademies.org/hmd/~/media/Files/Report%20Files/2001/Crossing-the-Quality-Chasm/Quality%20Chasm%202001%20%20report%20brief.pdf

King, C. R., & Gerard, S. (2016). *Clinical nurse leader: Certification review* (2nd ed.). New York, NY: Springer Publishing.

Maag, M. M., Buccheri, R., Capella, E., & Jennings, D. L. (2006). A conceptual framework for a clinical nurse leader program. *Journal of Professional Nursing, 22*(6), 367–372. doi:10.1016/j.profnurs.2005.11.002

Meleis, A. I., Sawyer, L. M., Im, E. O., Hilfinger Messias, D. K., & Schumacher, K. (2000). Experiencing transitions: An emerging middle-range theory. *Advances in Nursing Science, 23*(1), 12–28. doi:10.1097/00012272-200009000-00006

Moore, P., Schmidt, D., & Howington, L. (2014). Interdisciplinary preceptor teams to improve the clinical nurse leader student experience. *Journal of Professional Nursing, 30*(3), 190–195. doi:10.1016/j.profnurs.2013.09.013

Sheets, M., Bonnah, B., Kareivis, J., Abraham, P., Sweeney, M., & Strauss, J. (2012). CNLs make a difference! *Nursing, 42*(8), 54–58. doi:10.1097/01.NURSE.0000415837.20995.e2

Sotomayor, G., & Rankin, V. (2017). CNE Series. Clinical nurse leaders: Fulfilling the promise of the role. *MedSurg Nursing, 26*(1), 21–32.

CHAPTER

6 •••••

Nurse Educator Role

Gina M. Oliver

OBJECTIVES

1. Discuss the history of nursing education.
2. Compare and contrast the three major roles of the nurse educator.
3. Explain the three roles of an academic nurse educator.
4. Examine how a nurse educator can become nationally certified.
5. Distinguish the benefits and challenges of being a nurse educator.

All registered nurses have the responsibility for teaching patients and families. But as you earn your next professional degree, you may want to consider specializing in teaching and become a nurse educator.

HISTORY OF NURSING EDUCATION

Formal nursing education began in England with Florence Nightingale in hospital-based nursing programs. Nightingale used her knowledge acquired in Kaiserworth, Germany, to teach students the art and science of nursing. In Germany, she worked with Pastor Theodor Fliedner to learn the role of a deaconess who provided nursing care in hospitals (Attewell, 1998). It was after this experience that Nightingale wrote her book *Notes on Nursing* for the average housewife to provide nursing care in the home (Nightingale, 1969). Nightingale believed that nurses should be educated to nurse and not be handmaidens. She also believed strongly that nurses should be in charge of nursing as opposed to other disciplines such as medicine (Joel, 2011).

In the United States, a primitive nursing training program was initiated at New England Hospital for Women and Children in 1872. Students did not have any classwork, but rather worked from 5:30 a.m. to 9:00 p.m. every day in the hospital. Linda Richards is considered to be America's first trained nurse from this program in 1873, whereas Mary Mahoney is noted to be the first trained African American nurse in 1879 (Joel, 2011). The first three formal schools of nursing were established in 1873 at Boston Training School, Connecticut Training School, and Bellevue Training School (Dolan, 1975). These hospital-based diploma programs were based on the formal nursing education programs in England developed by Nightingale.

Baccalaureate degree programs in nursing began in 1909 at the University of Minnesota, which was the first university-based school of nursing (University of Minnesota School of Nursing, 2017). The baccalaureate degree ensured a well-rounded body of knowledge of the arts and sciences as well as essential nursing content. The initiation of the Yale School of Nursing in 1924 was a big step forward in nursing education as this was the first nursing program that was established as a separate university department with its own dean. This historic development was attributed to the Goldmark Report in 1923 that stated that nursing programs should be a separate unit or school within a university instead of a division of a similar unit such as a school of medicine (Gebbie, 2009).

Associate degree nursing programs originated in the early 1950s on the basis of a doctoral dissertation project written by Mildred Montag. Her project demonstrated how nurses could be educated in an accelerated manner down from 3 or 4 to 2 years to increase the number of nurses desperately needed to provide care during World War II (Montag, 1980). The intent of an associate degree was to educate a technical nurse who would provide care at the bedside as opposed to public health nursing or nursing management (Montag, 1963).

In the latter half of the 20th century, nursing programs moved toward increasing nursing knowledge. The American Nurses Association position paper in 1965 mandated that a baccalaureate was the minimal degree for entry into practice (Donley & Flaherty, 2008). In the 1970s, graduate education increased with master's degree programs primarily in nursing education and leadership. These programs were quickly followed by advanced practice areas of study including clinical nurse specialist and nurse practitioner. Prior to this time, nurses who wished to pursue doctoral education earned degrees in other disciplines such as education, sociology, psychology, and anthropology. The lack of doctoral programs in nursing led to the development of PhD programs in nursing as well as DNS and DNSc and the early practice doctorate in the ND (Ketefian & Redman, 2015). In 2004, the American Association of Colleges of Nursing (AACN) published the position statement regarding the practice doctorate, recommending that the Doctor of Nursing Practice be the standardized title for a practice doctorate and that all graduate degrees for advanced nursing practice preparation be at the doctoral level (AACN, 2004).

NURSE EDUCATOR ROLES

There are three major roles for a nurse educator: community educator, staff educator, and academic educator. Each role has a slightly different focus but uses the same basic skills taught in educator courses. First, a nurse educator must have knowledge of the faculty role as well as the content being taught. Next, faculty must have a good understanding of teaching skills, curriculum and course development skills, as well as evaluation and testing skills. Finally, faculty must have appropriate personal attributes to be an educator, such as attention to details, a love of lifelong learning, and a desire to assist others in meeting their educational goals (Bradshaw & Hultquist, 2017).

Community educators teach patients by increasing their knowledge and improving health outcomes. This education may be done with one patient at a time or in groups. Teaching in the community setting presents a unique set of issues to resolve, such as a patient's literacy level, varied knowledge levels, motivation and readiness to learn, cultural differences, language differences, and physiological barriers such as decreased vision or hearing. Community nurse educators learn to address these issues using multiple teaching strategies and individualizing the education as needed (Bastable & Alt, 2017).

Staff educators work in healthcare institutions and assist employees to provide safe and competent care through helping nurses to maintain and improve their knowledge base. Competencies may be assessed to determine where the learning needs are most needed and identify whether current practice standards are being implemented with patients and families. By improving nurses' knowledge, patient outcomes and satisfaction are improved (Bastable & Alt, 2017).

Academic educators work in collegiate settings in many levels. An academic educator typically has three major roles of teaching, research, and service. The extent to which faculty spend in each of these areas depends on the type and educational level of the academic institution as well as the type of faculty role, whether tenured or nontenured.

The Carnegie Classification of Institutions of Higher Education (2015) notes the type of collegiate institutions by degree level and program type. The degree level is primarily based on levels of education with undergraduate (associate and baccalaureate) versus graduate (master and doctorate). Educational institutions are also classified by public and private (nonprofit and profit). Universities with doctoral programs are then classified to the level of research intensity with moderate, higher, and highest. On the basis of these classifications, the academic institution will determine faculty roles by whether research and scholarship is required or a stronger focus on teaching is mandated. The institutional classification will also influence whether faculty will have the opportunity to be tenured or nontenured. The tenured process is primarily for faculty who teach but also have a program of research, whereas nontenured faculty focus on teaching (Fisher, 2016).

The academic educator roles of teaching, research, and service will vary between collegiate institutions but will definitely have similarities. The teaching role may consist of face-to-face or online didactic teaching, facilitating clinical practice, developing and grading assignments, and mentoring new faculty. Research and scholarly activities consist of implementing applied research that creates new nursing knowledge, taking the outcomes from applied research and doing translational research to see whether the results work in other settings, disseminating knowledge through presentations and publications, and applying for grant money to carry out new research. Service consists of committee work, student advising, working with student groups, participating in professional organizations, or being a leader in the nursing profession (Fressola & Patterson, 2017).

NURSING EDUCATION COMPETENCIES

The National League for Nursing (NLN) has developed a set of competencies for the academic nurse educator. Competencies reflect the basic knowledge and skills that all academic educators should reflect in the role.

These competencies include the following:

- Facilitate nursing

- Facilitate learner development and socialization

- Use assessment and evaluation strategies

- Participate in curriculum design and evaluation of program outcomes

- Function as a change agent and leader

- Pursue continuous quality improvement in the nurse educator role

- Engage in scholarship

- Function within the educational environment (NLN, 2012, p. 13)

The competencies show the breadth of an academic educator role and the variety of abilities needed to be an effective faculty member.

CERTIFICATION

Academic nurse educators may obtain national certification from the NLN to become a Certified Nurse Educator (CNE). Faculty may meet the criteria for taking the exam either by taking formal college courses related to nursing education or from on-the-job experience teaching in the collegiate setting. Successful completion of an online exam will result in becoming nationally certified for a span of 5 years. Faculty must renew the certification every 5 years by providing documentation that demonstrates expertise in the nursing education competencies (NLN, 2017).

ACCREDITATION

Academic educational institutions receive approval from the state board of nursing (SBON) from the state in which the school resides. This approval is required for the school to teach students in the selected state and notes how the school has met the minimum standards identified in the SBON rules.

Nursing school accrediting agencies began in 1950 with the NLN. Receiving accreditation is an optional process, although the majority of nursing schools choose to accept this process as it demonstrates that high quality of standards has been achieved. The accrediting arm of the NLN evolved into the National League for Nursing Accrediting Commission (NLNAC) and then into the Accreditation Commission for Education in Nursing (ACEN). The NLN broke the relationship with ACEN because of differences of opinion and developed a new subsidiary called the Commission for Nursing Education Accreditation (CNEA). The Commission on Collegiate Nursing Education (CCNE) is the autonomous agency that accredits schools of nursing that belong to the AACN.

FACULTY SHORTAGE

Currently, there is a significant shortage of nursing faculty in the United States. Many faculty are nearing retirement, and in the next 5 to 10 years, this shortage will be even greater (AACN, 2017). It is imperative that academic institutions strive to increase the number of master's degree and doctorate prepared faculty. Some organizations and many nursing schools are providing scholarship assistance for students earning a degree as a nurse educator. It is an excellent time to think about becoming a nurse educator.

BENEFITS AND CHALLENGE OF THE ACADEMIC NURSE EDUCATOR ROLE

Working as a nursing educator in the collegiate setting has many benefits. One significant advantage faculty have is the autonomy in coordinating their weekly schedule. Although nursing faculty must be present in the classroom and hospital when courses and clinicals are scheduled, the remaining hours in the week may be adjusted to fit the additional activities such as creating lectures, assignments, or exams; working on committee assignments; impacting public policy; or producing scholarly activities such as implementing research, presenting at conferences, or writing for publication. This autonomy also allows for significant creativity in teaching in choosing teaching strategies that are more student-centered and encouraging more active learning that is more true to real-life scenarios.

Additional benefits include maintaining a high level of current nursing knowledge and positively impacting the future of nursing. Faculty must keep updated on all health information used in the classroom and clinical setting to effectively facilitate student learning. Although this may take a bit of work, there is satisfaction in knowing that you are proficient in your field of expertise. There is also gratification in teaching others to provide quality healthcare. Although you may not be providing the care directly, you have educated students who will positively impact many lives. A final benefit as a faculty member is that you will never need to work on a major holiday ever again, very different from working as a staff nurse in the acute care setting.

As in any profession, there are challenges as an academic educator to consider. Teaching nursing is a not a standard 40-hours-per-week job. There may be weeks in which you will work beyond the norm to complete all necessary tasks, although this downside will be balanced with the extra weeks of vacation when school is not in session. In addition, the initial faculty salary is lower because of the majority of faculty contracts not including teaching during the summer session. Many faculty work part-time in the hospital setting to compensate for this difference in salary, with the added benefit of maintaining clinical competence while teaching.

Nursing education is an excellent role to consider when earning your master's degree. It provides flexibility in your work schedule and allows you to be at the top of the required knowledge in your area of expertise. As a nurse educator, you will impact many lives directly or indirectly. The personal gratification of seeing a patient or a student grow in his or her knowledge and positively impact healthcare, or mentoring a student to be a leader in the nursing profession, is heartening. As a nurse educator, you will make a difference in many lives.

CRITICAL THINKING QUESTIONS

1. Review the list of competencies for nurse educators published by the NLN. Which competencies do you feel strongly or excited about and which competencies make you nervous? Why do you think that is?

2. Discuss the value of obtaining and maintaining certification as a nurse educator.

3. Why do you think organizations such as CNEA, ACEN, and CCNE are important? How should schools of nursing choose which one to be accredited through?

4. Conduct a job search for faculty positions in your area. What kinds of jobs did you find? What are the requirements? How will your experience serve you in pursuing one of these positions?

REFERENCES

American Association of Colleges of Nursing. (2004). AACN position statement on the practice doctorate in nursing. Retrieved from http://www.aacnnursing.org/DNP/Position-Statement

American Association of Colleges of Nursing. (2017). Nursing faculty shortage fact sheet. Retrieved from http://www.aacnnursing.org/Portals/42/News/Factsheets/Faculty-Shortage-Factsheet-2017.pdf

Attewell, A. (1998). Florence Nightingale. *Prospects*, *28*, 153–166. doi:10.1007/BF02737786

Bastable, S. B., & Alt, M. F. (2017). Overview of education in health care. In S. B. Bastable (Ed.), *Nurse as educator: Principles of teaching and learning for nursing practice* (5th ed., pp. 3–30). Burlington, MA: Jones & Bartlett.

Bradshaw, M. J., & Hultquist, B. L. (2017). Effective learning: What teachers need to know. In M. J. Bradshaw & B. L. Hultquist (Eds.), *Innovative teaching strategies in nursing and related health professions* (7th ed., pp. 3–17). Burlington, MA: Jones & Bartlett.

Carnegie Classification of Institutions of Higher Education. (2015). 2015 update facts & figures: Descriptive highlights. Retrieved from http://carnegieclassifications. iu.edu/downloads/CCIHE2015-FactsFigures.pdf

Dolan, J. (1975). Nurses in American history: Three schools—1873. *American Journal of Nursing*, *75*, 989–992. doi:10.2307/3423429

Donley, S. R., & Flaherty, S. M. J. (2008). Revisiting the American Nurses Association's first position on education for nurses: A comparative analysis of the first and second position statements on the education of nurses. *Online Journal of Issues in Nursing*, *13*. doi:10.3912/OJIN.Vol13No02PPT04

Fisher, M. L. (2016). Teaching in nursing: The faculty role. In D. M. Billings & J. A. Halstead (Eds.), *Teaching in nursing: A guide for faculty* (5th ed., pp. 1–14). St. Louis, MO: Elsevier.

Fressola, M. C., & Patterson, G. E. (2017). *Transition from clinician to educator: A practical approach*. Burlington, MA: Jones & Bartlett.

Gebbie, K. M. (2009). 20th-century reports on nursing and nursing education: What difference did they make? *Nursing Outlook*, *57*, 84–92. doi:10.1016/j.outlook.2009.01.006

Joel, L. A. (2011). *Kelly's dimensions of professional nursing* (10th ed.). New York, NY: McGraw-Hill.

Ketefian, S., & Redman, R. W. (2015). A critical examination of developments in nursing doctoral education in the United States. *Revista Latino-Americana de Enfermagem*, *23*, 363–371. doi:10.1590/0104-1169.0797.2566

Montag, M. L. (1963). Technical education in nursing? *American Journal of Nursing*, *63*, 100–103. doi:10.2307/3452697

Montag, M. L. (1980). Looking back: Associate degree education in perspective. *Nursing Outlook*, *28*, 248–250.

National League for Nursing. (2012). *The scope of practice for academic nurse educators*. New York, NY: Author.

National League for Nursing. (2017). Certification for nurse educators. Retrieved from www.nln.org/professional-development-programs/Certification-for-Nurse-Educators

Nightingale, F. (1969). *Notes on nursing*. New York, NY: Dover Publications.

University of Minnesota School of Nursing. (2017). History. Retrieved from https://www.nursing.umn.edu/about/history

7

The Role of the Advanced Practice Nurse

Nycole Oliver

OBJECTIVES

1. Explain how the advanced practice nursing role was developed.
2. Compare and contrast the advanced practice nursing roles.
3. Examine theories used in advanced practice nursing roles.
4. Describe ethical issues impacting the advanced practice nurse (APN).
5. Apply ethics to the APN role.
6. Explore competencies of various advanced nurse practice roles.

Nurses have been viewed as caregivers since the inception of the occupation. Florence Nightingale established nursing as a profession in the mid-1800s during the Crimean War, and the importance of specialized training and education for nurses has subsequently been emphasized (Wilson, 2005). Since the early days of nursing, the scope and function of the profession have evolved significantly. Nurses originally performed with a great deal of autonomy, and in the 1960s, discussion began regarding developing the role even further because of the scarcity of primary care physicians (Wilson, 2005).

It became evident that knowledgeable, skilled professional nurses working in conjunction with physicians would make a positive impact on overall patient care (Silver, Ford, & Stearly, 1967). In response to the primary care shortage and in light of this realization, Dr. Henry Silver and Dr. Loretta Ford launched the initial nurse practitioner (NP) program at the University of Colorado in 1965. The progression of the occupation has resulted in over 234,000 NPs practicing today in multiple specialties (American Association of Nurse Practitioners [AANP], 2017c).

The purpose of this chapter is to discuss the history of the role, examine theories associated with the role, review ethical situations specific to the NP, assess organizations supporting NPs, explore competencies for NPs, and delineate information for individuals pursuing the NP designation.

HISTORICAL DEVELOPMENT OF THE ADVANCED PRACTICE ROLE

APNs encompass several clinical practice domains. The role has evolved because of the increasing demands of specific populations. Gaps between a specific need and practice were identified, and nurses were naturally chosen to fulfill the needs. Among the original APNs were nurse anesthetists, nurse-midwives, clinical nurse specialists, and NPs.

Nurse Anesthetists

The earliest APNs were nurse anesthetists, cultivated from development of anesthetics in the late 1800s. The task of administering anesthetics during surgery was originally delegated to nurses willing to administer the medications because the physicians were more intrigued with performing surgeries. Catherine S. Lawrence has been credited as the first nurse to administer anesthesia during the Civil War in 1863 (Ray & Desai, 2016). Alice Magaw ("Mother of Anesthesia") and Agatha Hodgins were among the most famous early nurse anesthetists. In the early 1900s, more formal education started for nurses wishing to pursue nurse anesthetist training (Ray & Desai, 2016). Subsequently, additional education and training were offered to the nurses, further developing the "advanced" role (Diers, 1991). The certified registered nurse anesthetist (CRNA) credential was realized in 1956 (Sipe, Fullerton, & Schuiling, 2009). Currently there are over 50,000 nurse anesthetists in practice in the United States (American Association of Nurse Anesthetists, 2016).

Nurse-Midwives

The next advanced practice role to develop was the nurse-midwife. The concept of midwifery has been documented since ancient times, but having a nurse acquire advanced training and knowledge to satisfy the role has been in effect only since the early 1900s (Savrin, 2009). In the early 1920s, Mary

Breckinridge traveled to England to learn midwifery with the intent of bringing the concept back to the United States. After her training, she chose a remote area in southeastern Kentucky and in 1925 founded the Frontier Nursing Service (FNS), originally named the Kentucky Committee for Mothers and Babies, which was proven to provide superior care (Schminkey & Keeling, 2015). Women sought encouragement during the birthing process, and the nurse-midwife was integrated into nursing practice (Sipe et al., 2009). As of August 2017, there are 11,826 Certified Nurse Midwives in the United States (American College of Nurse-Midwives, 2017).

Clinical Nurse Specialists

The next APNs were clinical nurse specialists. Clinical nurse specialists are APNs functioning as nurse clinicians within a specialty population. Discussions of the role development began in the early 1940s by Frances Reiter, and in 1954, Hildegard Peplau developed the first graduate-level psychiatric clinical nurse specialist program at Rutgers (Patten & Goudreau, 2012). The clinical nurse specialist designation was attained in the mid-1970s (Howard & Thorson, 2008). To date, there are over 72,000 clinical nurse specialists in practice in the United States using varying specialties, although a large number operate in tertiary centers (Explore Health Careers, 2017).

Nurse Practitioners

The final advanced practice role to mature was the NP. In the 1960s, a lack of primary care providers (because of physician specialization) and physician shortages, especially in rural areas, empowered Dr. Silver (pediatrician) and Dr. Ford (public health nurse) to explore options to fulfill the need. As a result of the rapidly increasing population and the lack of health services for children in particular, the original NP program was developed under collective support from the School of Medicine (Pediatric Department) and the School of Nursing at the University of Colorado in 1965 (Silver et al., 1967). The impetus of the program was to train professional nurses in managing ordinary childhood illnesses, as well as providing all-inclusive care for well-developing children (Wilson, 2005).

Studies revealed that patients felt care given by NPs was equal to care given by physicians, and since that time, the role has become more developed (Charney & Kitzman, 1971). By the 1980s, graduate degrees were required for NP practice. In 2003, a mandate for reduced work hours for medical residents by the Accreditation Council for Graduate Medical Education led to hospitals and other healthcare institutions hiring NPs in large numbers (Ralston, Collier, & Fairman, 2015). In 2008, a consensus model for APNs was developed in collaboration by the APRN Consensus Work Group and the National Council of State Boards of Nursing to help standardize training of APNs (Hartigan, 2011). A study performed by the AANP in 2017 concluded that over 234,000 NPs are licensed in the United States, an increase from the 222,000 in practice in 2016 (AANP, 2017c).

THEORY RELATED TO THE ADVANCE PRACTICE ROLE

Several theories, models, and philosophies for nursing are in existence. It is important for NPs to base the foundation of professional practice from these tools. Some specific theories and models are discussed in this section, including the following: Shuler's NP Practice Model, King's theory of goal attainment, Watson's theory of human caring, Benner's theory of novice to expert, and Mishel's uncertainty in illness theory.

Shuler's NP Practice Model

Pamela Shuler developed a model in 1991 for NPs because of the expanded role combining nursing (diagnosing and treating responses to actual or potential conditions) and medicine (diagnosing and treating conditions themselves). The Shuler NP Practice Model is wellness-oriented and provides a framework for how patient contact, assessment, intervention, and evaluation should transpire (Shuler & Davis, 1993). According to Shuler & Davis (1993), the impetus for the model is based on the following assumptions:

- People are physiological-psychological-social-cultural-environmental-spiritual beings.

- People have the right to refuse or accept care.

- The patient and the NP are partners in healthcare.

- Health is a dynamic state and wellness is an enduring process. Both are related to physiological, psychological, social, cultural, environmental, and spiritual characteristics of each patient.

- NPs support patients with wellness, maintenance, prevention, health promotion, and restoration through self-care activities.

- The NP is a role model for each patient and can influence the patient's health-related attitudes and behaviors.

- Patients can learn to move to an advanced level of wellness when facilitated by NPs who are well-rounded in wellness theory and practice.

- Family can be the paramount inspiration on the health behaviors of patients because health attitudes, beliefs, practices, and values are often regulated and monitored by this entity.

- Education regarding patient health can progress health and wellness status.

- One of the most significant roles of the NP is that of patient health educator.

- The patient is an active participant in the teaching/learning process.

- Learning needs and abilities vary throughout the life span.

The four concepts of the model are person, health, nursing, and environment, along with the NP role. The model is designed to guide NP practice and provide a framework for NPs to combine components of nursing and medicine, further defining the unique provider role (Shuler & Davis, 2013).

King's Theory of Goal Attainment

A nursing theory widely used today is Imogene King's theory of goal attainment. This theory was developed as a conceptual framework in the 1960s. The system exhibits collaboration of personal (perception, self, growth and development, body image, space, and time), interpersonal (interaction, communication, transaction, role, and stress), and social (organizational, authority, power, status, and decision making) systems (King, 1981; McQueen, Cockroft, & Mullins, 2017). She describes four concepts to form what she describes as the transaction process: perception, communication, interaction, and transaction. This process ideally could be used by the NP to incorporate the components of the nursing process in professional practice: assessing, diagnosing, planning, implementing, and evaluation of nursing care, as well as describing the interaction between the NP and the patient (King, 2007). King's theory can be beneficial and pertinent to current students and educators as it relates to the importance of communication, interaction, perception, stress, growth and development, personal space, and time in both work and personal lives (McQueen et al., 2017).

Watson's Theory of Human Caring

Jean Watson's nursing theory, Watson's Philosophy of Science and Caring, has four major concepts: health, human being, nursing, and environment/society. The model focuses on how nurses care for patients, and is outlined like the scientific process: assessment, planning, intervention, and evaluation. The model makes the following seven assumptions:

1. Caring can only be effectively validated and performed interpersonally.

2. Caring entails carative (as opposed to curative, as in medicine) aspects that result in human need gratification.

3. Successful caring promotes health and personal or family development.

4. Caring responses acknowledge the patients in their current state, as well as what they may become in the future.

5. An environment of caring is one that overtures the development of aptitude while allowing the patients to make decisions on their own behalf at a given point in time.

6. A science of caring is complementary to the science of curing.

7. The practice of caring is fundamental to nursing.

Watson developed 10 curative factors as a philosophical foundation for the model:

1. The formation of a humanistic–altruistic system of values, which allows the nurse to care for others in a selfless way.

2. The installation of faith–hope, which permits the nurse to honor the faith, hope, and belief systems of the self and others.

3. The cultivation of sensitivity to one's self and to others, which explores the need of nurses to feel an emotion as it presents itself.

4. The development of a helping–trust relationship, which includes compassion and warmth. This helps the nurse to listen, signifying empathetic understanding.

5. The support and acceptance of the expression of both positive and negative feelings, which helps the nurse and the patient understand the behavior it causes.

6. The systematic use of the scientific method for problem solving and decision making, which allows for direction and projection, and allows self-correction.

7. The promotion of teaching–learning opportunities, because the nurse should focus on the learning process as much as the teaching process.

8. The provision for a healing environment at all levels.

9. Assistance with healing–caring by attending to basic human needs.

10. Attending to the spiritual or existential unknowns of life or death. This helps the nurse assist the patient to find strength and courage during these inevitabilities (Petiprin, 2016b; Watson, 2008).

This nursing model is widely used today and can be used by APNs to incorporate the nursing process into individual practice.

Benner's Theory of Novice to Expert

Dr. Patricia Benner's theory of novice to expert is very commonly used in nursing practice to assess nurses' needs at the various stages of professional growth (Petiprin, 2016a). Benner's theory was originally developed from the Dreyfus Model of Skill Acquisition (developed by the Dreyfus brothers as a model for observing chess players, army commanders, Air Force pilots, and tank drivers) and applied it to nursing. She describes five stages of clinical competence:

- Novice
- Advanced beginner
- Competent
- Proficient
- Expert

Benner's theory proposes that skills and comprehension of patient care matures over time through appropriate educational backgrounds and personal encounters, further developing nurses as they progress through the five stages, culminating at the stage of expert (Benner, 1982; Petiprin, 2016a). This theory can also be applied to NPs as they progress through the five stages during their professional career.

Mishel's Uncertainty in Illness Theory

Another nursing model is Merle Mishel's uncertainty in illness theory. The theory addresses three components: antecedents of uncertainty, impaired cognitive appraisal, and handling uncertainty in illness (Mishel, 1981). Mishel (1981) states that the antecedents precede discernment of uncertainty of illness, and further subdivides them into the following: (a) stimulus frame, (b) cognitive capacities, and (c) structure providers. Dealing with real and/or perceived apprehensions and concerns regarding uncertainty experienced during illness is a significant characteristic of providing holistic care to patients and families during acute illness and hospitalization (Neville, 2003). Mishel's model can be applied to knowledge deficits regarding the NP role during acute illness and can help provide a framework for needs assessment and subsequent education and protocol development for the role.

Although several models and theories exist, it is important for the NP to be familiar with these frameworks to have a foundation on which to base professional practice. Only a few of the many theories, philosophies, and models have been discussed, and many more are in existence for the NP to explore.

ETHICAL ISSUES RELATED TO ADVANCE PRACTICE NURSING

Ethics is defined as a set of moral behaviors based on what is honorably correct or incorrect. NPs deal with special situations on a daily basis, and are faced with ethical decisions frequently. Ethical principles that can be encountered in the field of advanced practice nursing are the following: (a) nonmaleficence, (b) utilitarianism, (c) justice, (d) fidelity, (e) veracity, and (f) autonomy, among others. Each aforementioned principle is discussed in the following text with specific examples.

Ethical Principles

Nonmaleficence means that the APN is under obligation not to impose damage to others (Jahn, 2011). An example of nonmaleficence for the NP is ensuring that a patient has complete informed consent before performing any procedures on him or her, and making sure that the person is of a sound mind to make an informed decision about his or her care. Utilitarianism is doing the greatest good for the greatest number of people. This principle is particularly used in disaster triage, when limited resources are being used for a greater number of patients. Justice means equal distribution of resources (Jahn, 2011). In advanced practice nursing, justice is treating all patients equally and fairly, free of any bias.

Fidelity is based on the quality of caring and involves an agreement to keep a commitment or promise. The principle can be applied during end-of-life decisions as the APN respects the patient's wishes while supporting the family. Veracity is the concept of telling the truth (Regis University, n.d.). The NP could apply this principle during informed consent of a procedure, ensuring that the patient and/or family has complete information about the risks and benefits of the procedure, without any omissions or deception. Autonomy obligates the healthcare provider to respect the support of independent decision-making ability by the patient (Jahn, 2011). An example of autonomy is the right of the patient to have freedom of choice regarding treatments he or she chooses to partake in or refuse, if able.

Ethical Issues in Patient Care

An unexpected devastating injury or illness and the choices required for a patient at the time can have a deleterious effect on a patient's loved ones (Limehouse, Feeser, Bookman, & Derse, 2012). An advance directive can help ease the uncertainty and anxiety of decision making by loved ones during crucial moments by providing specific directions to a healthcare provider from the patient before incapacity (Limehouse et al., 2012). The two main types of advance directives are the power of attorney and living will. According to Limehouse et al. (2012), the power of attorney is an agent appointed by the patient to make healthcare decisions in the event the patient becomes debilitated and is unable to make decisions for himself or herself. A living will, on the contrary, is a document (without the use of an agent) stating what life-sustaining measures a patient wishes/does not wish to have in the event of a terminal condition (Limehouse et al., 2012).

Ethical Dilemma

An example of an ethical dilemma in patient care is the following: You have graduated NP school and are looking for a job. A popular family practice doctor likes your resume, and you do well in your interview. He decides to hire you. After orientation and a few weeks into practicing independently, you discover numerous people on your schedule who normally get narcotics and benzodiazepines monthly from your clinic, and have for several years. You attempt to stop prescribing the medications, but the patients are starting to get angry. One even states, "You are taking away medication that is keeping me alive." What do you do? Do you keep giving the patients their medications because they have been getting them from the physician all this time? Do you take a stand and wean the people on your schedule off their medications? Do you take all these people off your schedule and put them back on the physician's schedule? These and many other ethical dilemmas may arise during the course of the NP's career, and it is important for the NP to have a good understanding of different ethical principles to assist with solving these quandaries.

CERTIFICATIONS

Several NP certifications and certification boards exist, and it is important for the NP to have a good understanding of the options available, depending on the NP's education and training. It is also essential for the NP to be familiar with requirements in each state for board certification because not all states recognize certain boards/certifications. The following NP certifying bodies and certifications offered are discussed further: AANP, American Nurses Credentialing Center (ANCC), American Association of Critical-Care Nurses (AACN), Pediatric Nursing Certification Board (PNCB), and National Certification Corporation (NCC).

American Association of Nurse Practitioners

The AANP was founded in January 2013 as a merger of the American Academy of Nurse Practitioners (founded in 1985) and the American College of Nurse Practitioners (founded in 1995), forming the largest NP professional organization for all specialties (AANP, 2017b). It offers the following board certifications for NPs:

- Family Nurse Practitioner (FNP-C)

- Adult-Gerontology Nurse Practitioner (AGNP-C)

- Emergency Nurse Practitioner (ENP-C)

American Nurses Credentialing Center

The ANCC is a subsidiary of the American Nurses Association and was founded in 1990 (ANCC, 2017). It tenders the following NP board certifications:

- Adult-Gerontology Acute Care Nurse Practitioner (AGACNP-BC)

- Adult-Gerontology Primary Care Nurse Practitioner (AGPCNP-BC)

- Family Nurse Practitioner (FNP-BC)

- Pediatric Primary Care Nurse Practitioner (PPCNP-BC)
- Psychiatric-Mental Health Nurse Practitioner (PMHNP-BC)

American Association of Critical-Care Nurses

The American Association of Cardiovascular Nurses was founded in 1969 and changed the name in 1971 to the American Association of Critical Care Nurses (AACN, n.d.). This association has several board certifications for NPs, nurses, and Clinical Nurse Specialists, but only the NP board certifications are discussed here. The AACN has the following board certifications available at the advanced practice level for NPs:

- Acute Care Nurse Practitioner-Adult (renewal only; ACNPC)
- Adult-Gerontology Acute Care Nurse Practitioner (ACNPC-AG)

Pediatric Nursing Certification Board

The PNCB was established in 1975 and was called the National Certification Board of Pediatric Nurse Practitioners and Nurses. The name was changed in 2003 to the Pediatric Nursing Certification Board (PNCB, 2017). The following board certifications are available through PCNB for NPs:

- Primary Care Pediatric Nurse Practitioner (CPNP-PC)
- Acute Care Pediatric Nurse Practitioner (CPNP-AC)
- Pediatric Primary Care Mental Health Specialist (PMHS)

National Certification Corporation

The NCC was founded in 1975 to provide national certification in obstetric, gynecologic, and neonatal specialties (NCC, 2017). Board certifications for NPs offered through NCC are the following:

- Neonatal Nurse Practitioner (NNP-BC)
- Women's Health Care Nurse Practitioner (WHNP-BC)

ORGANIZATIONS SUPPORTING NURSE PRACTITIONERS

For NPs to continue to thrive in the profession, each individual has an ethical responsibility to become an involved member of at least one professional organization. Imagine the outcomes the profession would be able to accomplish if each NP (over 234,000 currently in practice) actively participated in professional organizations! NPs have several options, from organizations representing narrow specialties to organizations embodying more generalized roles. Even some medical specialty organizations have recognized the importance of the NP profession and have added membership categories for NPs (Goolsby & DuBois, 2017).

Professional organizations for NPs are vital for safeguarding and promoting the profession and role. Numerous organizations exist on the local, state, regional, national, and international levels supporting NPs and their unique specializations. The first NPs were prepared as pediatric NPs in 1965, so it comes as no surprise that the first NP professional organization to appear was the National Association of Pediatric Nurse Practitioners (NAPNAP). The next year, the National Organization of Nurse Practitioner Faculties (NONPF) was developed. (NONPF is discussed further in the section "Competencies for Nurse Practitioners.") The next associations to develop were in women's health, followed by gerontology. In 1985, the American Academy of Nurse Practitioners was founded (now the AANP) to include NPs of all specialties (Goolsby & DuBois, 2017).

Not only do NP organizations have benefits for the profession but most have individual benefits also. Continuing education, advocacy resources, conferences, mentoring programs, grants and scholarships, association journals, special interest groups, and mentoring programs are among the several benefits offered (ANCC, 2017; AACN, 2017; AANP, 2017b; PNCB, 2017; NCC, 2017). Many organizations even offer a student membership at a reduced rate.

COMPETENCIES FOR NURSE PRACTITIONERS

In 1990, the NONPF identified core competencies for all NPs. The competencies represent the minimum level of practice required on graduation from an NP program. In 2017, the NONPF released the most current, nationally validated set of core competencies for NPs (NONPF, 2017). Population-focused competencies are also available through the NONPF in collaboration with specialty-focused organizations. The core competencies encompass several areas, including the following:

- Scientific foundation
- Leadership
- Quality
- Practice inquiry

- Technology and information literacy
- Policy
- Health system delivery
- Ethics
- Independent practice (NONPF, 2017)

Each of these core competencies is further subdivided into specific objectives, which are examined in more detail in the following text.

The NP should base decisions using nursing and scientific theory, and progress advanced practice by critically examining data and evidence and transforming the knowledge obtained into nursing practice. APNs are expected to stay up-to-date on the latest evidence-based guidelines and incorporate them into the everyday nursing practice when seeing patients. In using the latest guidelines and nursing theory, NPs are enhancing patient outcomes (DeCapua, 2014; NONPF, 2017).

NPs have a unique role in leadership. In healthcare, multiple stakeholders are involved in patient care, and NPs can use critical thinking skills to collaborate with all members involved in patient care to improve outcomes. The NP is responsible for practicing in the most cost-effective manner without compromising care. Again, NPs have a professional obligation to maintain knowledge on the most current guidelines in order to provide the best possible care for each patient, as well as to retain membership in professional organizations. Professional organizations assist with networking between NPs in similar practice areas and allow members to share ideas and practice innovations (DeCapua, 2014; NONPF, 2017).

The NP should be able to consider how different changes through policy, marketing, finance, and organizational structure can affect patient care. Changes are inevitable, and the NP can adapt and transform practice on the basis of change. The NP can tailor care for each patient on the basis of the most current evidence-based guidelines, and should encourage a culture of excellence through a peer review process (DeCapua, 2014; NONPF, 2017).

The NP should continually seek out knowledge and disseminate it to others in the field. Researchers are constantly coming up with new methods for practice, and the NP is in a perfect position to analyze and apply the new methods when caring for patients. The NP has a unique set of clinical experiences to assist with development of practice and can improve patient outcomes by collaborating with other NPs to determine the paramount treatment for any given ailment (DeCapua, 2014; NONPF, 2017).

Technology is continuously changing, and it is important for NPs to keep up with modern information systems to promote safe, high-quality, cost-effective patient care. Many practices use tablets to keep up with patient records, check patients in, and show patients the latest treatments in medicine. Other practices use telemedicine and other similar methods to care for patients from a distance. The author personally encourages the use of applications for patients to keep up with changes in health, weight, calories, vital signs, blood sugars, and so on (DeCapua, 2014; NONPF, 2017).

Policies in relation to healthcare are perpetually under review, and it is vital for the NP to stay current with any changes affecting NP practice. NPs also have a professional duty to keep in contact with policy makers and advocate for advancement of the role to better serve the patient population in their area. The APN should understand the implication of global issues on health policy and practice and campaign for safe practice environments (DeCapua, 2014; NONPF, 2017).

The NP is always looking for ways to make healthcare better and should use critical thinking skills for improvement. Collaboration with other professionals as well as any stakeholders involved in patient care is crucial to be able to prompt necessary changes across the continuum of care. The NP must analyze resource allocation and organizational structure to improve delivery of healthcare and reduce provider and patient risk (DeCapua, 2014; NONPF, 2017).

The NP should use ethical principles discussed earlier when making decisions in clinical practice. Many ethical situations can arise in practice and the NP is duty-bound to analyze and apply ethical significance of choices in practice. Each population is different, and the NP must take each specific population and their needs into consideration when making clinical decisions (DeCapua, 2014; NONPF, 2017).

NPs practice at different levels depending on the state. Currently, 23 states in the United States grant full practice authority to NPs. This authorization means NPs in the respective states can evaluate and diagnose patients, as well as order and interpret diagnostic tests and manage treatments, including medications, without a collaborative practice agreement with a physician (AANP, 2018). The ability to practice to the full extent of the NP has been realized in the 23 states because of the relentless efforts of NPs in the states advocating and campaigning for independent professional practice (DeCapua, 2014; NONPF, 2017).

APNs learn to use advanced assessment skills to deliver the full spectrum of healthcare services, and distinguish between normal and abnormal assessment findings. Depending on the state, NPs can prescribe a variety of medications, including controlled substances, while managing the healthcare of patients and families over the life span. It is also important for NPs to provide culturally competent care, taking into consideration each unique patient and his or her cultures/beliefs.

IMPORTANT INFORMATION

Although the role of the APN has developed in a major way, there is still much work to be done. It is important for APNs to continually seek out educational opportunities to further progress their own performance and stay up-to-date with the most current guidelines for NP practice. NPs are encouraged to join professional organizations to further develop and advocate for the role. It is also crucial for the NP to stay enlightened on legislation related to the occupation and advocate for progression of the role.

In 2010, the Institute of Medicine recognized a need and placed a formidable recommendation that APNs be able to practice to the full scope of training and advocated that barriers to full practice be removed (Stewart, 2013). With that mandate, NPs should be dignified to make forward progress for the profession. As of 2017, a total of 23 states in the United States have full practice authority for NPs (AANP, 2017a). This accelerative movement has happened because of the tireless work of NPs and NP advocates campaigning and promoting the role.

This chapter has assessed the history of the NP role, described theories associated with the role, examined ethical situations specific for NPs, reviewed organizations supporting NPs, investigated competencies for NPs, and appraised information for individuals pursuing the NP designation.

CRITICAL THINKING QUESTIONS

1. Identify certifications for an advanced practice role of your choice.

2. Locate the competencies for an advanced practice role other than the NP and discuss how they compare with those of a NP.

3. Visit the Bureau of Labor Statistics (www.bls.gov) and search for each of the identified advanced practice roles in this chapter. What is the anticipated growth rate over the next 5 to 10 years? How do growth rates for each of the roles compare with one another? Do you think there is a connection between them?

4. Explore liability insurance options for the advance practice roles identified in this chapter. How do the costs compare? Why do you think that is?

REFERENCES

American Association of Critical-Care Nurses. (2017). Clinical Resources. Retrieved from https://www.aacn.org/clinical-resources

American Association of Critical-Care Nurses. (n.d.). Complete history of AACN. Retrieved from www.aacn.org

American Association of Nurse Anesthetists. (2016). Certified registered nurse anesthetists fact sheet. Retrieved from https://www.aana.com/membership/become-a-crna/crna-fact-sheet

American Association of Nurse Practitioners. (2017a). Nurse practitioner state practice environment. Retrieved from https://www.aanp.org/legislation-regulation/state-legislation/state-practice-environment

American Association of Nurse Practitioners. (2017b). About AANP. Retrieved from www.aanp.org

American Association of Nurse Practitioners. (2017c). National nurse practitioner database. In *NP Facts*. Retrieved from https://www.aanp.org/all-about-nps/np-fact-sheet

American Association of Nurse Practitioners. (2018). State practice environment. Retrieved from https://www.aanp.org/legislation-regulation/state-legislation/state-practice-environment

American College of Nurse-Midwives. (2017). Midwives and births in the United States. Retrieved from http://www.midwife.org/Essential-Facts-about-Midwives

American Nurses Credentialing Center. (2017). About ANCC. Retrieved from www.nursecredentialing.org

Benner, P. (1982). From novice to expert. *American Journal of Nursing, 82,* 402–407. doi:10.2307/3462928

Charney, E., & Kitzman, H. (1971). The child-health nurse (pediatric nurse practitioner) in private practice: A controlled trial. *New England Journal of Medicine, 285*(24), 1353–1358. doi:10.1056/NEJM197112092852405

DeCapua, M. (2014). What are the nurse practitioner core competencies? Retrieved from https://www.nursepractitionerschools.com/faq/what-are-the-np-core-competencies

Diers, D. (1991). Nurse midwives and nurse anesthetists: The cutting edge in specialist practice. In L. H. Aiken & C. M. Fagin (Eds.), *Charting nursing's future: Agenda for the 1990's* (pp. 159–180). New York, NY: Lippincott Williams & Wilkins.

Explore Health Careers. (2017). Clinical nurse specialist. Retrieved from https://explorehealthcareers.org/career/nursing/clinical-nurse-specialist/

Goolsby, M. J., & DuBois, J. C. (2017). Professional organization membership: Advancing the nurse practitioner role. *Journal of the American Association of Nurse Practitioners, 29*(8), 434–440. doi:10.1002/2327-6924.12483

Hartigan, C. (2011). APRN regulation: The licensure-certification interface. *AACN Advanced Critical Care, 22*(1), 50–65. doi:10.1097/NCI.0b013e3182072684

Howard, J. C., & Thorson, M. A. (2008). Society of Trauma Nurses position statement on the role of the clinical nurse specialist in trauma. *Journal of Trauma Nursing, 15*(3), 91–93. doi:0.1097/01.JTN.0000337148.21926.71

Jahn, W. T. (2011). The 4 basic ethical principles that apply to forensic activities are respect for autonomy, beneficence, nonmaleficence, and justice. *Journal of Chiropractic Medicine, 10*(3), 225–226. doi:10.1016/j.jcm.2011.08.004

King, I. M. (1981). *A theory for nursing: Systems, concepts, process.* Albany, NY: Delmar.

King, I. M. (2007). King's conceptual system, theory of goal attainment, and transaction process in the 21st century. *Nursing Science Quarterly, 20*(2), 109–116. doi:10.1177/0894318407299846

Limehouse, W. E., Feeser, V. R., Bookman, K. J., & Derse, A. (2012). A model for emergency department end-of-life communications after acute devastating events–Part I: Decision-making capacity, surrogates, and advance directives. *Academic Emergency Medicine, 19*(9), E1068–E1072. doi:10.1111/j.1553-2712.2012.01426.x

McQueen, L., Cockroft, M., & Mullins, N. (2017). Imogene King's theory of goal attainment and the millennial nurse: An important mentoring tool for nurse educators. *Teaching and Learning in Nursing, 12*(3), 223–225. doi:10.1016/j.teln.2017.03.003

Mishel, M. H. (1981). The measurement of uncertainty in illness. *Nursing Research, 30,* 258–263.

National Certification Corporation. (2017). About NCC. Retrieved from https://www.nccwebsite.org/about-ncc.aspx

National Organization of Nurse Practitioner Faculties. (2017). Nurse practitioner core competencies content. Retrieved from https://www.nonpf.org/page/14?&hhsearchterms=%22core+and+competencies+and+content%22

Neville, K. L. (2003). Uncertainty in illness: An integrative review. *Orthopedic Nursing, 22*(3), 206–214. doi:10.1097/00006416-200305000-00009

Patten, S., & Goudreau, K. A. (2012). The bright future for clinical nurse specialist practice. *Nursing Clinics of North America, 47*(2), 193–203. doi:10.1016/j.cnur.2012.02.009

Pediatric Nursing Certification Board. (2017). About us. Retrieved from www.pncb.org

Petiprin, A. (2016a). From novice to expert. Retrieved from http://www.nursing-theory.org/theories-and-models/from-novice-to-expert.php

Petiprin, A. (2016b). Jean Watson nursing theory. Retrieved from http://www.nursing-theory.org/theories-and-models/watson-philosophy-and-science-of-caring.php

Ralston, B., Collier, T. H., & Fairman, J. (2015). The NP: Celebrating 50 years. *American Journal of Nursing, 115*(10), 54–57. doi:10.1097/01.NAJ.0000471941.77288.a4

Ray, W. T., & Desai, S. P. (2016). The history of the nurse anesthesia profession. *Journal of Clinical Anesthesia, 30,* 51–58. doi:10.1016/j.jclinane.2015.11.005

Regis University. (n.d.). Ethics at a glance: Veracity. Retrieved from http://rhchp. regis.edu/hce/ethicsataglance/Veracity/Veracity_01.html

Savrin, C. (2009). Growth and development of the nurse practitioner role around the globe. *Journal of Pediatric Health Care, 23*(5), 310–314. doi:10.1016/j.pedhc.2008.10.005

Schminkey, D. L., & Keeling, A. W. (2015). Frontier nurse-midwives and antepartum emergencies, 1925 to 1939. *Journal of Midwifery & Women's Health, 60*(1), 48–55. doi:10.1111/jmwh.12212

Shuler, P. A., & Davis, J. E. (1993). The Shuler nurse practitioner practice model: A theoretical framework for nurse practitioner clinicians, educators, and researchers, part 1. *Journal of the American Academy of Nurse Practitioners, 5*(1), 11–18. doi:10.1111/j.1745-7599.1993.tb00835.x

Silver, H. K., Ford, L. C., & Stearly, S. G. (1967). A program to increase health care for children: The pediatric nurse practitioner program. *Pediatrics, 39*(5), 756–760.

Sipe, T. A., Fullerton, J. T., & Schuiling, K. D. (2009). Demographic profiles of certified nurse-midwives, certified registered nurse anesthetists, and nurse practitioners: Reflections on implications for uniform education and regulation. *Journal of Professional Nursing, 25*(3), 178–185. doi:10.1016/j.profnurs.2009.01.002

Stewart, J. G. (2013). The nurse practitioner: Historical perspectives on the art and science of nurse practitionering. In J. G. Stewart & S. M. DeNisco (Eds.), *Role development for the nurse practitioner* (pp. 1–34). Burlington, MA: Jones & Bartlett.

Watson, J. (2008). *Nursing: The philosophy and science of caring* (Rev. ed.). Boulder, CO: University Press of Colorado.

Wilson, K. (2005). The evolution of the role of nurses: The history of nurse practitioners in pediatric oncology. *Journal of Pediatric Oncology Nursing, 22*(5), 250–253. doi:10.1177/1043454205279288

SECTION III

Indirect Care Roles

The previous section reviewed the direct care roles. This section focuses on the indirect care roles held by the master's-prepared nurse. All master's-level nursing roles have an impact on patient care and outcomes. However, you may be asking yourself what makes some direct and some indirect. While indirect care roles have an impact on patient care and outcomes, their functions may not include direct physical contact with patients. Although this list and chapter are not inclusive of all indirect roles, we are focusing on those highlighted by the American Association of Colleges of Nursing (AACN; see Table 2.1 in Chapter 2).

CHAPTER 8

Public Health Nurse

Brenda Scott and Dana Hill

OBJECTIVES

1. Define public health.
2. Compare and contrast public health and community health.
3. Describe the 10 essential public health services.
4. Examine the ethical considerations of the public health nurse.
5. Describe the research opportunities available to nurses for specialization within public health.
6. Identify organizations committed to advancing nursing and public health.
7. Evaluate certifications available to nurses practicing public health.

The role of a nurse is multifaceted. Nurses have many career opportunities, many of which do not consist of hospital bedside nursing. Each nursing pursuit has significance and leaves a handprint on society and the health of populations. Nurses often become nurses because they perceive this career as a "calling" of sorts. For many, the draw to nursing begins with a sense that there needs to be care in the world. This care can involve the hands-on care of bringing new life into the world, or hand-holding of the dying, to everything in between. This is where public health nursing lies—in the in-between. This chapter begins by defining what public health nursing means. Information is also presented on the history, theories, ethical situations, certifications, supporting organizations, and competencies for this unique nursing role of caring for the public.

WHAT IS PUBLIC HEALTH?

Typically, when people think of public health nursing, they think of the nurses they see at their local health department. There are dozens of facets of public health nursing that involve more than the nurses working at county health departments. Public health is a type of care involving a reduction of disease at a level of the population, rather than at the individual level. Public health is an organized effort to prevent disease occurrence, treat maladies, teach the public about sanitation and health practices, control outbreaks, protect people from environmental hazards, and serve communities for the health and well-being of all in the community (Novick, Morrow, & Mays, 2008).

Public health is a science and an art. The science lies in the knowledge of the research regarding best practices in disease prevention and the reliance on epidemiological data to guide education and practice. The art of public health is a bit more subjective, as the art of public health involves building relationships and trust with the public to assess and meet the needs of individuals in the community and to persuade individuals to adhere to the common health needs for populations (Turnock, 2006). Persuasion is not always about moving individuals toward common goals of population health (such as immunizations or quarantines), but involves the development and successful implementation of public policy. When public policy is made, there must also be effective means of communication of the policy to engage the community and vie for community support and adherence to protective policies and laws (Clark, 2015).

Everyone may be considered a member of the public at large, so it is somewhat difficult to define public health in terms that specify the difference between individual and population health. It may be thought of in a generalization of medicine as being the treatment of disease or illness and public health as being a focused effort for the prevention of disease. In county health departments, this line may seem blurred as individuals are diagnosed and treated for some illnesses, such as sexually transmitted diseases; however, many illnesses are treated in a physician's clinic, urgent care clinic, or emergency department (ED; Clark, 2015; Schneider, 2006).

Another difference between individual medicine and population medicine is how funding occurs and how politics have an influence on funding and practice issues in the public health arena. In practices involving the treatment of individuals, physicians charge a fee and are paid on the basis of private or public insurance (such as Medicaid and Medicare). Medicaid and Medicare are controlled by politics and public tax-based funding; however, physicians may choose to refuse treatment of individuals on the basis of ability to pay if Medicaid or Medicare funding is no longer available (Clark, 2015). The current climate in the United States is rocky for the continuation of public funds in many sectors of public healthcare. With the advent of the Affordable Care Act (ACA), multiple aims were set in motion for the care of the public and for disease prevention. The fifth aim of the ACA specifically addressed the need for an expansion in preventative care at the community level (Rosenbaum, 2011). In 2017, Donald Trump became the president of the United States with a platform of a promise to repeal the ACA. Many physicians, leaders, and citizens believe that such a repeal would put Americans at risk for a loss in healthcare as public funding for healthcare initiatives and insurance would be diminished or no longer exist (Oberlander, 2017).

You may have also heard about community health. This is a branch within public health. McKenzie, Pinger, and Kotecki (2005) define community health as "the health status of a defined group of people and the actions and conditions, both private and public (governmental), to promote, protect, and preserve their health" (p. 5). Simply stated, community health is the delivery of care on the basis of public health needs. This delivery would be the more direct care roles within public health. Although you may often hear these two terms used interchangeably, they really are two separate roles. We discuss roles of the public health and community health nurses later in the chapter.

HISTORY OF PUBLIC HEALTH

How did we get to where we are today with public health? The famous story about John Snow is usually one of the first stories that come to mind when students consider the beginning of public health. In 1854, Mr. Snow investigated an outbreak of cholera and found the source to be the town water pump—the source of drinking water for citizens in the town (Jardim, 2015). Once the source of infection was discovered, Mr. Snow had to convince citizens to avoid the use of this water source. When students think of public health nursing, they may think of Florence Nightingale. In 1854 (the same year Mr. Snow found the source of the cholera outbreak), Nightingale and a team of 38 other nurses attended to the needs of war victims of the Crimean War. During her time there, Ms. Nightingale put the nurses to work sanitizing the "wards" of the hospital and decreased mortality rates from 32% to just 2% during her 3 years (Winkelstein, 2009).

There are hundreds of stories, which could be told, regarding the start of public health, but these two demonstrate three very important aspects of public health. First, Mr. Snow and Ms. Nightingale *recognized* there was a problem affecting a group or population of people. Second, each of them observed the situation, calculated incidence rates, and went on an investigative hunt to find the source of the disease transmission or occurrence.

Finally, Mr. Snow and Ms. Nightingale courageously *advocated for* and *acted to* communicate their findings and to stop disease proliferation. These two individuals demonstrated necessary characteristics of leaders and partners in the public health workforce.

NURSING AND PUBLIC HEALTH

Nursing in public health is multidimensional. In the past two decades, public health leaders have sought to define specific functions of public health. These started with the document "The Future of Public Health" published in 1988 by the Institute of Medicine. By the early 1990s, the core functions morphed into the "10 Essential Functions of Public Health." Further revisions occurred in 2010, whereas the essential functions became a reflection of eight domains of core competencies of public health. The core competencies (Centers for Disease Control and Prevention [CDC], 2017) consist of the following:

- Policy development

- Analytical assessment

- Knowledge of public health sciences

- Competency in cultural differences

- Communication

- Practice at the community level

- Management and financial planning

- Leadership and "systems" thinking

These core competencies were developed with the intention of building on these skills to enhance and implement the 10 essential functions of public health. In 2014, further revisions were made to the essential functions and the core competencies to better meet the challenges of health needs and prevention needs and initiatives. The current "10 Essential Public Health Services" include the following (CDC, 2017, p. 1):

1. Monitor health status to identify and solve community health problems.

2. Diagnose and investigate health problems and health hazards in the community.

3.   Inform, educate, and empower people about health issues.

4.   Mobilize community partnerships and action to identify and solve health problems.

5.   Develop policies and plans that support individual and community health efforts.

6.   Enforce laws and regulations that protect health and ensure safety.

7.   Link people to needed personal health services and assure the provision of healthcare when otherwise unavailable.

8.   Assure a competent public and personal healthcare workforce.

9.   Evaluate effectiveness, accessibility, and quality of personal and population-based health services.

10. Research for new insights and innovative solutions to health problems.

The core competencies were changed to reflect specific recommendations for Tier 1, Tier 2, and Tier 3 public health workers. These core competencies became a part of the Healthy People 2020 Objectives for all pieces (essential functions, core competencies, healthy people goals) to work in concert and support the overall initiatives of bringing better health to populations (CDC, 2017).

As a public health nurse, your focus is on each of these 10 essentials. If you were to pull a job description of a public health nurse, you will likely find the essentials weaved throughout the position requirements. Although these essentials are primarily the focus of the public health nurse, almost all nursing roles focus on one aspect or another.

Prevention

Much of the public health nurse's role focuses on prevention. Whether it is working in a health department or in occupational health, the primary focus is prevention. This is no different than most other specialties within nursing; we are all focused on prevention. Within public health, this attention to prevention is heightened. Remember the public health nurse is focused on the whole population versus one individual patient. This is the primary difference.

Ethical Considerations

There are ethical considerations within public health nursing just as with any other branch of nursing. Some may say the ethical situations arise more frequently in public health. No matter which area of nursing you work in, your goal as a nurse is to protect the patients and their privacy. In public health, you are not just concerned with protecting the individual patient, but rather the whole population becomes your focus.

Commonly, communicable diseases are at the forefront when considering public health. Can you imagine the ethical dilemmas that may arise when dealing with this very sensitive topic? As a nurse, there are certain diseases that must be reported to the CDC. It is important to be aware of the reporting structure within the facility in which you work. If you are a nurse working in the county health department, you may be responsible for reporting. In many hospital settings, the reporting of required diseases occurs within the laboratory department or the infection prevention department. From time to time, facilities rely on the CDC to confirm diagnoses with diagnostic testing at remote laboratory settings. Again, determination of the reporting structure is one aspect of patient care where you will want to ensure processes are followed.

Even with communicable disease reporting, it is the responsibility of all involved to maintain patient or population privacy. There are times where this can cause an ethical dilemma. Consider the following: You are providing care for a 20-year-old female who was recently diagnosed with chlamydia. During your interview, she reveals she has had two partners within the past 2 weeks. You know the importance of treating all contacts. How will you go about contact notification? Many health departments have an anonymous partner notification process. You can give the patient the option to tell both contacts to seek treatment or to provide the contact information for the nursing staff to notify. If provided the contact information, you must ensure patient privacy is maintained while protecting the health of the public. Can you see how this might create an ethical dilemma? When notifying the contact, you may be asked who gave you their name. You legally cannot provide this information.

Another ethical situation that may arise in public health is during mass prophylaxis. One recent example was the H1N1 influenza (flu) outbreak of 2009. Because this was a strain of the flu never seen before, initially the vaccine was unable to be produced at a rate fast enough to immunize all members of the population. The decision was made to vaccinate those at the greatest risk first. Once more vaccine became available, the greater population was offered the vaccination (CDC, 2010). Can you see how this could create an ethical dilemma for nurses?

SPECIALTIES WITHIN PUBLIC HEALTH AND COMMUNITY HEALTH NURSING

There are several specialties within public health. As we discussed earlier, community health is a branch of public health. We review several public and community health specialties in this section. Although this list is comprehensive, it is not all-inclusive.

Epidemiology

One primary function of the public health nurse is the focus of epidemiology. According to the CDC (2012), the definition of epidemiology is

> the study (scientific, systematic, data-driven) of the distribution (frequency, pattern) and determinants (causes, risk factors) of health-related states and events (not just diseases) in specified populations (patient is community, individuals viewed collectively) and the application of (because epidemiology is a discipline within public health) this study to the control of health problems.

Nurses work in a variety of positions that focus on epidemiology. Even bedside nurses, not working specifically in public health nursing, are concerned with many aspects of epidemiology.

When a disease outbreak occurs, the epidemiology specialists are commonly involved. The team is usually made up of an epidemiologist, nurses, and other healthcare professionals. Their primary focus is to determine the distribution and determinants of the outbreak. There are a lot of fact-finding processes that occur as a part of the outbreak investigation. Outbreak investigation is just one small example of the role of the nurse in epidemiology.

Disaster and Emergency Preparedness and Response

Have you ever been in a situation where your local healthcare system has been overwhelmed because of a lack of resources? What about where not only the local healthcare system has exhausted all resources but also the city/county/state/territory is completely overwhelmed? What did you do? How did you continue to perform your role? How would you do it during a pandemic? Do you remember the fear and panic from H1N1? Many people think of catastrophic events such as major hurricanes and life-changing tornadoes, but do not realize there are disasters and emergencies that occur every day. The World Health Organization (2002) defines a disaster as "an occurrence disrupting the normal conditions of existence and causing a level of suffering that exceeds the capacity of adjustment of the affected community." In the United States, an emergency management cycle is used to look at disasters. This cycle consists of five phases: preparedness, prevention, mitigation, response, and recovery.

Preparedness and Prevention

The nurses' involvement in disaster might depend on which phase of the cycle they are participating in. One of the key elements of disasters is preventing their occurrence and being prepared when they do occur. As a nurse, one way to increase preparedness and prevention is educating patients on reducing risky behaviors that can lead to preventable disasters and emergencies. Nurses can also volunteer with organizations such as the American Red Cross, Save the Children, National Safety Council, Medical Reserve Corp, local injury prevention coalitions, and other organizations to educate children and the public as to the dangers of fire and local disasters that place their communities at risk. Another way nurses can be involved in the first three phases is participation in local emergency planning, legislative and policy development and support, and an overall understanding of the challenges of the impact of disaster both domestic and internationally. Nurses can also practice preparedness by understanding their facilities' emergency operation plan (what to do, where first aid kits are, automated external defibrillators, safe rooms, etc.), participating in facility exercises, and knowing what to do personally when the time comes.

Response and Recovery

In terms of response and recovery, there are numerous ways that nurses can participate. As an master's-prepared nurse, individuals will look to you to manage and lead during times of crisis. One of the first ways nurses participate in disaster response is by being prepared to make a mental shift. Knowing that the local healthcare system is going to be impacted, nurses must be prepared to transition from normal daily activity to whatever is required for the scope and duration of the disaster or emergency. Practicing a disaster response using your facility's emergency operation plan will prepare you for when you are called to lead. With this comes an understanding that surge is likely and that nurses will not be able to provide care for every single patient who requires it. Disaster triage will be necessary, and some tough decisions are likely. Often, resources will be in high demand and short supply.

Nurses must be familiar with local plans and able to function under the incident command system or hospital incident command system. (Your local protocols will dictate the appropriate courses; however, training in both is recommended.) This education can be obtained through the

U.S. Federal Emergency Management Administration and your local facility. Nurses can also participate in domestic and international response activity through a variety of organizations that are both members and nonmembers of voluntary organizations active in disaster (VOAD), state and federal response programs such as the U.S. Public Health Service, National Disaster Medical System, Medical Reserve Corps, and more. During disasters, nurses may be asked to serve in a variety of healthcare facilities, shelters, and alternative care and practice sites.

Following a disaster, the return to normalcy as safely and quickly as possible is the goal. This return is called recovery. In recovery, nurses can help to serve as a voice and advocate, monitor the short-term and long-term physical and emotional needs and well-being of the population, and push for change. Recently, the American Nurses Credentialing Center (ANCC) released a disaster certification for nurses and other healthcare professionals called the National Healthcare Disaster Professional Board Certification (NHDP-BC; ANCC, 2018b). This certification requires training, participation in disaster exercises, and the completion of a national standardized computer-based examination.

Occupational and Environmental Health Nursing

Since its birth, the United States has been a country that set out to make it on its own. This attitude was found and felt in everything including the progression and industrialization of the country. With the growth in industrialization, the number of workers employed in hazardous areas such as factories, coal mines, textile plants, oil and metal refineries, and others increased. During this growth period, occupational nursing began to emerge. One of the first recorded engagements of nurses in occupational health comes from Pennsylvania in 1888 (American Association of Occupational Health Nurses [AAOHN], 2018). During this time, a nurse named Betty Moulder provided care for coal miners and their families (2018). Throughout the next decades, nurses' help would be required to increase workplace cleanliness, prevent the spread of infectious disease, and provide immediate treatment for workers (2018). Over the years, the United States' industrial base has shifted, but that does not mean manufacturing is no longer important.

Did you know that in 2013, approximately 9% of the U.S. workforce was employed in manufacturing (Scott, 2015)? In the Midwest and South, this number rises significantly. Despite aggressive laws, safety standards, process revisions, and methods to make the work safer, it remains dangerous work. In many of these manufacturing and food production facilities, nurses help as part of, and often leaders of, occupational and environmental health programs. For these nurses, the multiple facets of their jobs include case management, counseling, health promotion, hazard reduction, physical examinations, immunizations, hearing tests, drug and alcohol testing, accident investigation, rendering emergency aid, treating chronic pain, and much more. Often, these nurses hold master's degrees in nursing, public health, advanced practice, safety, and other related professional areas (AAOHN, 2018).

Occupational and environmental health nurses are represented through multiple organizations and associations, and although there are many organizational certifications available, there are two primary certifications, both from the American Board for Occupational Health Nurses: the Certified Occupational Health Nurse (COHN) and the Certified Occupational Health Nurse-Specialist (COHN-S). The COHN certification is focused on direct care roles and primarily for clinicians, whereas the COHN-S is more appropriate for those with managerial and programmatic roles and responsibilities. Although both exams are computerized exams, it is highly recommended that the nurses choose the exam that plays to their knowledge base, skills, and abilities (Association of Occupational Health Professionals in Healthcare, 2018).

Correctional Nursing

As you might recall, in the United States the legislative branch creates and adopts laws. The judicial branch is responsible for enforcing the law. With criminal activity being a routine occurrence, a portion of the population is incarcerated and in the custody of local, state, or federal government authorities for breaking the established rules of this country. Carson (2018) found that more than 1.5 million people were in federal or state custody in 2016. Although these individuals are incarcerated, their well-being is the responsibility of the government. To make sure these individuals remain healthy, nurses are employed within many facilities across the country.

Because of the very nature of the population being housed, each facility is considered an individual community. As an individual community, these facilities are faced with many challenges associated with the well-being of the individual. Nurses in correctional facilities often wear many hats and must problem-solve issues with other medical and nonmedical team members. Some of the challenges correctional nurses might be faced with include the following: ensuring the environment within the facility is sanitary and not conducive to the spread of infectious diseases, surveillance of disease outbreaks, providing case management to prisoners with chronic health issues, and providing routine and emergency care to patients with acute and chronic illness and traumatic injury. This specialty is not for every nurse and requires a nurse to see the patient and not the crime or circumstances that are present. This specialty requires a nurse to always be aware of safety and security risk and protocol. Nurses must also be mentally prepared for the environment they will be working inside.

It is recommended that a nurse achieve traditional nursing experience before entering correctional nursing. For nurses practicing in a correctional setting, certification as a Certified Correctional Healthcare Professional (CCHP) is available through the National Commission on Correctional Healthcare (National Commission on Correctional Healthcare, 2018). At present, the CCHP is a certification that applies to many occupations within corrections following the completion of a national computerized exam and all set requirements. Upon achieving certification as a CCHP, nurses in corrections may then apply and test for a specialty as a CCHP-RN.

Military Nursing

Another specialty within public health nursing is the nursing task of ensuring the well-being of armed forces service members and their dependents domestically and across the globe. Many current medical processes are rooted in practice adapted from the military. Some of the most famous nurses, such as Florence Nightingale, Clara Barton, Jane Delano, Florence Blanchfield, Mary Walker, and even the nurse and poet Walt Whitman, were civilians contributing to military service. In 1901, the U.S. Army took its understanding of the need for nurses a step farther and established the U.S. Army Nursing Corps (U.S. Army Medical Department Office of Medical History, 2014). This corps allowed nurses to serve and hold military rank.

Today military nurses have completed their Registered Nurse, all the requirements for enlisting and commissioning by their specific branch of armed forces (Army, Air Force, Navy [provide medical care for Navy, Marine, and Merchant Marine personnel], and Coast Guard), and typically have a specialty certification like those of their civilian counterparts. The nurses serving in the nurse corps are often master's or doctorally prepared. Because of the unique structure of military service, these nurses may find themselves serving in a variety of roles and specialties and supervising other nurses and non-nursing healthcare professionals (medic/corpsman, other paramedical professionals, administrative personnel, etc.).

Depending on the branch of service, rank, and assignment, the nurses can find themselves in charge of programs with few nurses or service members to thousands. These nurses serve in a variety of settings including clinics, hospitals, surgery units, mobile medical facilities, ships, helicopters, aircraft, and more. For those in this setting, the focus around public health centers on a healthy military and their dependents. Maintaining the health of the specific population is achieved through prevention, surveillance, epidemiology, and chronic and emergency medical care.

School Nursing

When parents send their children to school, there is a transferal of responsibility and care. During this time, parents expect school staff to be trained, ready, and equipped to handle whatever may occur from small everyday issues to wide-scale disaster. Although some may not consider school nursing as part of public health nursing, the focus as with the other specialties we have identified is to provide care within a specific community.

School nursing traces its roots back to New York City and 1902 when nurse Lina Rogers was hired to reduce student absence because of diseases (National Association of School Nurses, Inc. [NASN], 2017). School nurses play a huge role in disease surveillance, prevention, preparedness, case management, and more. They are involved in leading school districts through changes and growth to health services provided within school systems (Maughan, Bobo, Butler, & Schantz, 2016). School nurses also play a large role in community disease and injury prevention by providing education on topics such as sexually transmitted diseases, smoking cessation, healthy weight, and more. In this way, the school nurse brings together communities around education, health, and healthcare over the school career of students (NASN, 2017).

Organizations

When it comes to nursing in general, but specifically public health nursing, it is important for the nurse to be a part of shaping the future. One way that nurses can do this is through the participation in organizations dedicated to public health. There are two major organizations in the United States committed to public health: the Association of Public Health Nurses (APHN) and the American Public Health Association (APHA).

Although reorganized in 2012, the APHN traces its roots back to the Association of State and Territorial Directors of Nursing (ASTDN) in 1935 (APHN, 2018). The ASTDN served as an advisory council made up of state health department nurses. Today, the APHN is organized and committed to being advocates for and advancing public health nursing. The APHN has also worked to build a toolkit for public health advocacy and to be part of the development of public health competencies. It also offers monthly newsletters, annual conferences, and continued education to improve public health nursing across the United States (APHN, 2018). There are also career listings and public health forums for members to communicate through.

The second organization is the APHA. The APHA, although not strictly nursing focused, is a 145-year-old organization devoted to improving public health through improvements to a variety of professions and issues across the country (APHA, 2018). The association is also a nationally recognized organization that is responsible for publishing the *American Journal of Public Health* and the *Nation's Health* (2018). The APHA has multiple member sections that are sector and occupationally specific that allow members to present, share, and discuss public health issues impacting their communities. It also asks its members to engage in political advocacy by sharing issues and the APHA position with elected officials and through the support of multiple public health awareness campaigns.

Certifications

In any profession, including public health nursing, it is important to be able to demonstrate competency and expertise through knowledge, skills, and experience. Current and future employers and professionals at large know the importance of becoming certified in a field and look for demonstrated excellence. There are two specific certifications that may be of interest to nurses practicing in public health: the ANCC's Advanced Public Health Nursing certification and the Certification for Public Health (CPH).

The ANCC certification is a 5-year certification formally called the Advanced Public Health Nursing Board Certification (PHNA-BC; ANCC, 2018a). This certification requires candidates to submit a portfolio demonstrating experience, education, and training in four primary domains: professional development, professional and ethical nursing practice, teamwork and collaboration, and quality and safety (ANCC, 2018a). As part of this portfolio, peer and self-evaluations must also be performed.

The CPH is the second primary certification offered. With the CPH, education and experience are weighted and used to determine eligibility. The goal of the CPH is to determine whether a candidate has the knowledge, skills, and abilities to meet the 10 essential public health services defined by the CDC (National Board of Public Health Examiners [NBPHE], 2018). Once eligibility has been determined, a candidate will be invited to take either the computerized examination or a proctored written exam. Once granted, recertification is required per NBPHE requirements.

SUMMARY

This chapter covers several types of public health nursing. The primary focus of most nurses is prevention. The key to avoiding major public health concerns is to prevent them in the first place. When nurses are unable to prevent health concerns, they need to be prepared to respond. Nurses have many opportunities to teach their patients and communities about prevention and preparedness.

CRITICAL THINKING QUESTIONS

1. What is one way you function as a public health nurse in your current practice? Identify how this relates to public health.

2. Are you prepared for disaster? If not, what steps do you need to take to become prepared?

3. What are three things you learned from this chapter?

4. How can you adapt your practice to focus more on prevention?

REFERENCES

American Association of Occupational Health Nurses. (2018). History. In *What is occupational & environmental health nursing?* Retrieved from http://aaohn.org/page/profession-of-occupational-and-environmental-health-nursing

American Board for Occupational Health Nurses. (2016). ABOHN certification programs. Retrieved from https://www.abohn.org

American Nurses Credentialing Center. (2018a). Advanced public health nursing portfolio. Retrieved from https://www.nursingworld.org/our-certifications/advanced-public-health-nurse

American Nurses Credentialing Center. (2018b). National healthcare disaster certification. Retrieved from http://www.nursecredentialing.org/Certification/NurseSpecialties/National-Healthcare-Disaster-Certification

American Public Health Association. (2018). About APHA. Retrieved from https://www.apha.org/about-apha

Association of Occupational Health Professionals in Healthcare. (2018). Certifications. Retrieved from http://aohp.org/aohp/EDUCATION/Certifications.aspx

Association of Public Health Nurses. (2018). APHN's history. Retrieved from http://www.phnurse.org/APHNs-Story

Carson, E. A. (2018). Prisoners in 2016. In *Publications and products: Prisoners, January 2018 NCJ 251149*. Retrieved from https://www.bjs.gov/content/pub/pdf/p16.pdf

Centers for Disease Control and Prevention. (2010). The 2009 H1N1 pandemic: Summary highlights, April 2009-April 2010. Retrieved from https://www.cdc.gov/h1n1flu/cdcresponse.htm

Centers for Disease Control and Prevention. (2012). Lesson 1: Introduction to epidemiology. In *Principles of epidemiology in public health practice* (3rd ed.). Retrieved from https://www.cdc.gov/OPHSS/CSELS/DSEPD/SS1978/Lesson1/Section1.html#_ref1

Centers for Disease Control and Prevention. (2017). The public health system and the 10 essential public health services. Retrieved from https://www.cdc.gov/stltpublichealth/publichealthservices/essentialhealthservices.html

Clark, M. (2015). *Population and community health nursing* (6th ed.). [Bookshelf Online]. Retrieved from https://bookshelf.vitalsource.com/#/books/9780133943979/

Jardim, J. B. (2015). John Snow's behaviorsphere. *Psychological Record, 65*(1), 209–213. doi:10.1007/s40732-014-0082-3

Maughan, E. D., Bobo, N., Butler, S., & Schantz, S. (2016). Framework for 21st century school nursing practice: National Association of School Nurses. *NASN School Nurse, 31*(1), 45–53. doi:10.1177/1942602X15618644

McKenzie, J. F., Pinger, R. R., & Kotecki, J. E. (2005). Community health: Yesterday, today, and tomorrow. In J. A. Mark, J. C. Bolduc, & N. Quinn (Eds.), *An introduction to community health* (p. 5). Sudbury, MA: Jones & Bartlett.

National Association of School Nurses. (2017). The role of the 21st century school nurse. Retrieved from https://schoolnursenet.nasn.org/blogs/nasn-profile/2017/03/13/the-role-of-the-21st-century-school-nurse

National Board of Public Health Examiners. (2018). CPH FAQs. Retrieved from https://www.nbphe.org/cph-exam-faqs/

National Commission on Correctional Health Care. (2018). Advance your career, gain personal satisfaction, become certified. Retrieved from https://www.ncchc.org/professional-certification

Novick, L. F., Morrow, C. B., & Mays, G. P. (2008). *Public health administration: Principles for population-based management*. Sudbury, MA: Jones & Bartlett.

Oberlander, J. (2017). The end of Obamacare. *New England Journal of Medicine, 376*, 1–3. doi:10.1056/NEJMp1614438

Rosenbaum, S. (2011). The Patient Protection and Affordable Care Act: Implications for public health policy and practice. *Public Health Reports, 126*(1), 130–135. doi:10.1177/003335491112600118

Schneider, M. (2006). *Introduction to public health*. Sudbury, MA: Jones & Bartlett.

Scott, R. E. (2015). The manufacturing footprint and the importance of U.S. manufacturing jobs. Retrieved from http://www.epi.org/publication/the-manufacturing-footprint-and-the-importance-of-u-s-manufacturing-jobs/

Turnock, B. (2006). *Public health: Career choices that make a difference*. Sudbury, MA: Jones & Bartlett.

U.S. Army Medical Department Office of Medical History. (2014). The Army Nurse Corps: More than 111 years of selfless service to our nation; embracing the past—engaging the present—envisioning the future. In *About the Army Nurse Corps*. Retrieved from http://history.amedd.army.mil/ancwebsite/about.html

Winkelstein, W., Jr. (2009). Florence Nightingale: Founder of modern nursing and hospital epidemiology. *Epidemiology, 20*(2), 311. doi:10.1097/EDE.0b013e3181935ad6

World Health Organization. (2002). Disasters & emergencies: Definitions. Retrieved from http://apps.who.int/disasters/repo/7656.pdf

CHAPTER 9

MSN as Informaticist

Ellie Hunt

OBJECTIVES

1. Describe different nursing informatics (NI) roles.
2. Compare the informatics competencies of a nurse, informatics nurse, and informatics nurse specialist (INS).
3. Examine theories used in NI.
4. Describe the legal issues impacting informatics.
5. Apply ethics to the role of informatics in practice.

WHAT IS NURSING INFORMATICS?

NI is a nursing specialty formally recognized in 1992 by the American Nurses Association (ANA). Informatics nurses are expert nurses with analytical and critical thinking skills. Over the years, nurses have increasingly moved into this specialty. The ANA's second edition of *Nursing Informatics: Scope and Standards of Practice* (2014) states:

> *Nursing Informatics (NI) is the specialty that integrates nursing science with multiple information and analytical sciences to identify, define, manage, and communicate data, information, knowledge, and wisdom in nursing practice. NI supports nurses, consumers, patients, the interprofessional healthcare team, and other stakeholders in their decision-making in all roles and settings to achieve desired outcomes. (pp. 1-2)*

The first scope of practice was published in 1994, followed by a combined scope and standards in 2001 and revised in 2008. Then in 2014, the second edition of the scope and standards of practice for NI was released (ANA,

2014; McGonigle & Mastrian, 2014). Advances in knowledge and information management have been incorporated and the definition of NI has changed slightly to include multiple information and analytical sciences including computer, information, cognitive, library, archival, information management, and the science of terminologies and taxonomies.

An informatics nurse very often acts as the bridge between clinical care and the information technology department. The nurse will advocate for both nursing and the patient in an area where most of the focus is on technological solutions. Informatics nurses make sure technology does no harm, improve clinical and quality reporting, eliminate redundancies in data collection, and make an effort to capture nursing data to prove nursing's inherent value in patient outcomes (Sensmeier, 2012).

The focus of informatics nurses includes supporting the decision making of the interprofessional care team by synthesizing data and information into knowledge and wisdom (ANA, 2014). NI supports data analytics, and informatics nurses understand that real-time application of accurate information is vital to improving patient outcomes. It promotes data integrity and the access and exchange of health data, supports interoperability, and incorporates key ethical concerns such as advocacy, privacy and confidentiality, and security of data and information (ANA, 2014). Like all nurses, informatics nurses ensure that collaboration is an integral part of practice, and consider the impact of technological changes on healthcare delivery, quality reporting, patient outcomes, and nursing practice (ANA, 2014).

How Is That Nursing?

Similar to other indirect roles in nursing, such as nurse manager or case manager, an informatics nurse most often provides support to the staff who provide direct care to patients. If you think of the patient in the center of a set of concentric circles, the direct care staff take care of immediate needs (Figure 9.1). Indirect care staff provide the direct care staff with the support needed for the best care of the patient. The organization then provides the support to all staff caring for the patient.

Informatics nurses support patient care in several ways, which includes standardizing documentation via the electronic health record, applying information management techniques to the data gathered, being an expert in process re-engineering, and contributing to research and evidence collection (Sensmeier, 2012).

Another way to think of the informatics role is to consider that many decisions made on a daily basis directly affect the care provided to hundreds, if not thousands, of patients. For example, changing the options in a charting

FIGURE 9.1 Visual Representation of how Nursing Informatics Supports Patient Care Indirectly.

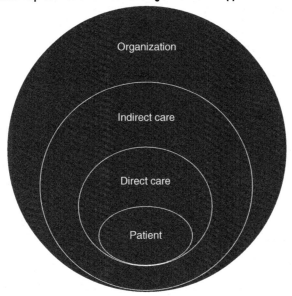

pathway such as the admission assessment is not something that should be done quickly or without thought. That is why approvals are required before an update goes into use. Interprofessional committee work is vital to the informatics nurses to ensure that correct information and decisions are being implemented.

NURSING INFORMATICS ROLES

Common Roles

Common NI roles include help desk support, analyst, manager, director, and chief nursing informatics officer (CNIO; Hunt, Sproat, & Kitzmiller, 2004). Consider the help desk support and analyst roles as similar to a staff nurse role. That is the role that is closest to the system and system users. In either of those roles, the informatics nurse typically interacts with end users and recommends or makes the changes that end users see. The manager role includes making sure there are adequate analysts for the work, providing guidance on priorities, and being involved in meetings to ensure that NI is represented (Hunt et al., 2004). The director provides guidance to the managers, and the CNIO is at the executive level, similar to the level of chief nursing officer (CNO) or chief nursing executive (CNE). You will also find informatics nurses in areas or roles in education as faculty, training as trainers, project management, consulting, policy development, and more.

Common Work Settings

Informatics nurses work in a variety of care settings including acute care, ambulatory care, long-term care, home health, hospice, dialysis centers, schools, and corporate offices of health systems. In addition, you might find nurses working for information technology vendors such as EHR vendors, medical device vendors, as well as insurance companies. You might also find informatics nurses in professional organizations and local, state, or federal agencies. Essentially, wherever you find direct care nurses, you will probably also find informatics nurses.

Educational Preparation

Typically, the INS role is assigned to a registered nurse with formal graduate-level education. Although a diploma-, associate's-, or bachelor's-prepared registered nurse will be called an informatics nurse (ANA, 2014), in practice, the job titles of nurses working within informatics tend to be a bit messy and are not uniformly applied across the board. This means that, in practice, nurses tend to continue to use their credentials and their job title in their signatures.

PROFESSIONAL ORGANIZATIONS

The Alliance of Nursing Informatics (ANI) brings together thousands of informatics nurses by bridging the various workgroups, committees, councils, or sections within them. It is a great starting point to find an organization local to you or that matches your interests. For example, some state nurse's associations have councils specific to NI, such as the North Carolina Nurses Association's Council on Nursing Informatics. Check out which meetings are most actively attended in your area, and join one.

The Healthcare Information Management Systems Society (HIMSS) has an NI committee, taskforce, and subgroups. HIMSS also has an NI symposium each year at the annual HIMSS conference. The American Medical Informatics Association (AMIA) is the academic association and has a nursing informatics working group (NIWG). Other professional organizations also have NI committees, subgroups, taskforces, or specialty assemblies, such as the Association for Perioperative Registered Nurses (AORN). A good starting point for more research is the ANI website's listing of member organizations.

CERTIFICATIONS

There are several certifications that informatics nurses commonly obtain. The American Nurses Credentialing Center (ANCC) has a Nursing Informatics Specialty exam that provides the credential RN-BC. The professional organization HIMSS offers entry-level and specialist-level informatics certifications (CAHIMS and CPHIMS). Product management and project management certifications such as PMP and PgMP are also common for nurses developing products or managing projects. If the nurse is in the executive realm, such as a CNIO, he or she might also obtain Nurse Executive certifications.

How Do I Enter the Informatics Specialty?

There are several ways to enter the specialty, and each usually hinges on gaining experience or allowing you to demonstrate experience. Once you gain experience and contacts, start to look for positions and apply. A degree or certification in informatics is not necessarily required, depending on how the job description is written. If a job description is written with a degree or certification requirement, talk to the hiring manager about your interest. Many times, the most important part of the position is the clinical aspect and the technology can be learned.

Many informatics nurses enter the specialty by initially volunteering for technology-related projects, implementations, or committee work, or by becoming a credentialed trainer and training nurses new to the organization. Other ways to gain experience include joining one or more professional organizations and volunteering on workgroups or committees. Volunteering could take the form of writing white papers, working on standards, or otherwise lending your clinical expertise to a technology project. Another idea to generate contacts, obtain continuing education, and widen your knowledge is to volunteer to coordinate continuing education sessions specific to informatics in your local area. The experience gained from volunteering will add to your resume.

If you are thinking about obtaining certification from either HIMSS or ANCC, look at the requirements. Consider the costs of continuing education requirements needed for renewal, and how long a certification will last. As mentioned earlier, a common path to entering the specialty is to obtain a degree or post-master's certificate in the specialty. Often the requirements of either of these journeys involve reaching out to those working in information technology or doing a project. Working toward certification grows your experience and contacts.

NURSING INFORMATICS COMPETENCIES

In 2008, a joint task force identified basic informatics competencies that all healthcare professionals need to support their daily practice. All healthcare professionals need to be competent in the areas of privacy, confidentiality, and security related to technology, skilled in using an electronic health record, have basic computer literacy skills, and have health information literacy and skills (McGonigle & Mastrian, 2014).

In 2010, the Technology Informatics Guiding Education Reform (TIGER) initiative published a report outlining informatics competencies for every practicing nurse that incorporated informatics into undergraduate and graduate curriculum. In 2017, this report was updated to be an interprofessional, interdisciplinary document and incorporated the international standards being adopted across healthcare. These competencies are available free for anyone to read at HITComp.org. Use the filters to narrow the competencies to baseline, basic, intermediate, advanced, and expert for different domains (HITComp, 2017).

THEORY RELATED TO ROLE

Common theories used in NI include the metaparadigm that describes NI practice and change theories, including Lewin's theory and Roger's Diffusion of Innovation. It is also important to consider nursing theories in conjunction with technology so that we do not lose the *caring* aspect of nursing, even though technology is being increasingly incorporated into practice.

The overarching metaparadigm has been used in NI since 1989 and is the idea of data-information-knowledge-wisdom (Graves & Corcoran, 1989; Ronquillo, Currie, & Rodney, 2016). Now known as the D-I-K-W metaparadigm, it is not unique to NI but has driven the direction of informatics for some years now (Ronquillo et al., 2016). Essentially, informatics nurses work to help make sense of an overwhelming amount of data, turn the data into information, generate knowledge, and then wisdom. This D-I-K-W metaparadigm was originally represented as a pyramid (see Figure 9.2), concentric circles, cones, or even a flowchart (McGonigle & Mastrian, 2014; Ronquillo et al., 2016).

Nurses use Lewin's Theory of Change all the time in NI. They often use it to implement new technologies, or perhaps use it in conjunction with Rogers Diffusion of Innovations theory. Lewin's change theory works well for informatics to assist with the concept of breaking the bonds to the old technology, making the change to the new technology, and then providing a level of support to solidify the new technology into new practice. "By using Lewin's theory, [nurses] can help reduce stakeholder resistance and

FIGURE 9.2 Data-Information-Knowledge-Wisdom (D-I-K-W) Metaparadigm.

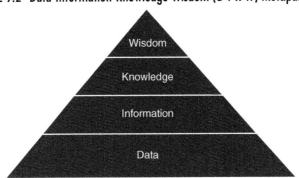

fear of change through the development of a well thought plan and active participation in the change process" (Sutherland, 2013, p. 2).

Rogers Diffusion of Innovations is used to understand how the diffusion of technology often works and leverage that knowledge in implementation planning. In essence, once the innovators, early adopters, and early majority are on board with using the technology, the tide has turned and it is inevitable that the late majority will come along. The bell curve of how innovations get adopted also means that there are laggards, who may never fully adopt the technology, and there are strategies to use to make sure those laggards do not negatively impact the adoption of technologies (Hunt et al., 2004).

For staff being on the receiving end of the technology, there is usually not a lot of choice involved, but preparing the staff and anticipating the change, making the change, and then freezing that new technology and workflow in place by conducting an evaluation is a method often used. These are not all the theories used, but hopefully give a flavor of the types of theories used to frame NI practice.

LEGAL ISSUES

HIPAA

Most nurses have heard of the Healthcare Information Portability and Accountability Act (HIPAA) that was originally passed in 1996. Did you also know that the Health Information Technology for Economic and Clinical Health (HITECH) Act of 2009 strengthened HIPAA to include *electronic* personal health information (ePHI)? With all the changes to HIPAA over the years, the Office for Civil Rights (OCR) released the HIPAA omnibus in 2013 that gathered together all the pieces and parts of HIPAA.

So now, if you are interested in seeing what HIPAA is all about, you can start with the 2013 omnibus and continue with updates from that point on.

There are three parts to HIPAA: the privacy rule, the security rule, and the breach notification rule. The privacy rule is a set of federal standards aimed at protecting the privacy of patients' medical records and other health information (U.S. Department of Health & Human Services [DHHS], 2017a). It covers health information that is maintained by covered entities that include health plans (both private plans and federal plans such as Medicaid, Medicare, and the VA), doctors, hospitals, many other healthcare providers, and healthcare clearinghouses as well as any business associates (DHHS, 2017b). It also defines patients' rights to view and correct their medical records.

The security rule is another set of standards that ensures the security of electronic protected health information (PHI; DHHS, 2017c). The breach notification rule requires that breaches of unsecured PHI be quickly reported, and provides instructions on how to report breaches (DHHS, 2017a). Most organizations have a security officer position that can be called on if there are any questions or concerns about HIPAA.

Informatics nurses need to be generally aware of HIPAA requirements and include the security officer on anything involving privacy, security, or a potential breach of information. PHI includes any information that can identify a patient and his or her health diagnosis or condition, provision of healthcare, or payment of healthcare (DHHS, 2015). Demographics alone are not considered PHI (e.g., phone book listings are fine), but when they are associated with health information, demographics become PHI.

Licensure

Informatics nurses need to be aware of several licensure concerns. The first concern is knowing the licensure requirements of nurses in your particular state. You will be amazed at what nurses might consider as part of their role, when they might actually be operating outside of their license. Every board of nursing has someone you can talk to if you need to clarify what is within an LPN, RN, and APRN practice. For example, licensure becomes relevant to the informatics nurse when he or she is training, setting up the role requirements within a system, or documenting workflow.

Another licensure concern occurs when you are near a state line or if you are supporting any telehealth applications. The National Council of State Boards of Nursing have information about the extended Nursing Licensure Compact (eNLC). Keep an eye on the list of states that are part of the eNLC, which allows nurses to provide care to patients in other eNLC states without having to obtain additional licenses (National Council of State Boards of Nursing, 2017).

Social Networking

Because a nurse is responsible for protecting a patient's privacy and confidentiality, nurses need to be very aware of what they post to social media. Social media could include any application that allows individuals to create a profile and share information online. Social media is a great way to network with colleagues, provide ways to express feelings, keep up to date with industry trends, and see other points of view. However, there are pitfalls associated with social media, as well. All nurses need to understand the boundary between personal and professional life and adhere to their organization's social media guidelines. Check the organization's employee handbook for guidelines to avoid inappropriate use of social media. The ANA has a social networking principles toolkit available for all nurses to use. The tooklit's guidelines recommend that nurses refrain from discussing patient information online, stay within ethical patient–nurse boundaries when considering social media, comprehend social media's reach, and understand that information cannot be recalled once sent or posted (ANA, n.d.).

ETHICAL SITUATIONS SPECIFIC TO ROLE

In addition to HIPAA, did you know that the ANA Code of Ethics for Nurses mandates that nurses protect a patient's rights to privacy and confidentiality? This code means that a registered nurse cannot turn a blind eye to privacy being breached.

CASE STUDY

You are part of a project that is implementing provider order entry to ambulatory practices in a rural community. While training front desk staff at a medical practice, the intake nurse comes in and sits at a side desk to return a patient's phone call. The intake nurse connects the call, asks for the patient by first and last name, and continues with the call, asking detailed health questions and confirming the details of the conversation while writing down notes. As you look out in the relatively full waiting room, you wonder how much of the conversation could be audible to the waiting room patients. Because you are aware of HIPAA privacy rules, you quietly speak to the

practice manager about a better location for the intake nurse to be returning phone calls. The practice manager realizes your concern and takes
immediate steps to ensure PHI is not being potentially shared in an open
area. The practice manager identifies another area that the intake nurse
can use to return phone calls, located in the medical records section, which
provides an area away from patients who could overhear conversations.

Alternate Action

If the practice manager had not taken immediate action or did not appear to
listen, what steps could you have taken next? If your organization has a security officer, you could phone or email your concern to the office and he or she
could conduct a privacy and security audit of the practice. Alternatively, you
could speak to the practice owner to share your concerns. You could mention
to the practice owner that any patient could file a breach notification, and that
could incur significant civil penalties. You could ask the practice owner if he
or she knows the ins and outs of the HIPAA rulings and provide the number
of your organization's security officer to clarify any questions or concerns.

JOINING THE SPECIALTY

If this specialty interests you, then join us! If your organization uses an
electronic health record, see if there are committees or opportunities to
volunteer to learn a bit more. There might be an opportunity to become a
credentialed trainer and teach an orienting class each month or so. That is
a great way to get your foot in the door, get to know the informatics team,
and be considered for any opportunities that arise.

Reach out to a fellow informatics nurse and ask whether he or she would
mentor you as you pursue your interest. I would also encourage you to read
the ANA Nursing Informatics Scope and Standards of Practice for further
details on what the specialty does and does not do (ANA, 2014). Consider
joining a professional organization or start to read healthcare information and
management news. Share your interest with your immediate manager so that as
committee appointments or opportunities arise, your name can get forwarded.

PROFILE

Jane Both, MSN, RN-BC
Jane started her career as a bachelor's-prepared nurse, graduating from
New York University. Her current role is Director of Clinical Informatics
at a regional medical center. Jane worked as an NICU nurse for the first

12 years of practice. She advanced in her practice, but shared that she never had the opportunity to be in leadership.

Feeling that she needed to grow and needed a change, Jane decided to make a lateral move to a similar position, but in a very different environment with a slightly different population. Jane started to work in home care with an at-home baby program where she visited Medicaid moms with newborns. While at the home care company, Jane also volunteered for stretch projects such as data and quality reporting and a new technology rollout plan for respiratory techs.

By volunteering for extra projects, Jane developed skills that were outside of her current position. This experience led to her subsequent positions. For example, the home care laptop program extended to nurses was a success. Jane did such a great job with that project, the CNO of the associated community hospital asked her to come back to a hospital setting to implement barcode scanning for meds. Jane then moved to working as a data quality and safety analyst, and then moved into a director of education and research position. While in this position, Jane decided to go back to school and earned her master's in nursing. The organization was going to implement CPOE but she moved to another state.

Jane first wanted to work where she works now, but there were no positions available, so she took a job at a very small community hospital. She waited for a position to open where she really wanted to work, and quickly applied when one became available and worked her way up in that organization, again volunteering for committees and opportunities that were related to data, informatics, and technology. For example, in a patient safety position, she volunteered for the CPOE project, and then moved into an informatics analyst position when one was created.

CRITICAL THINKING QUESTIONS

1. What did you learn about the informatics role that surprised you?

2. Informatics is a term often not fully understood. Explain your understanding of what informatics is and how it is used in healthcare.

3. Is informatics a specialty you can see for yourself? Why or why not?

4. Discuss your experience working with informatics teams. If you have not worked in an organization with an informatics team, how do you imagine such a team would collaborate with other healthcare staff?

REFERENCES

American Nurses Association. (n.d.). Social networking principles toolkit. Retrieved from https://www.nursingworld.org/practice-policy/nursing-excellence/social-networking-Principles/

American Nurses Association. (2014). *Nursing informatics: Scope and standards of practice* (2nd ed.). Silver Spring, MD: Author.

Graves, J. R., & Corcoran, S. (1989). The study of nursing informatics. *Journal of Nursing Scholarship, 21*(4), 227–231. doi:10.1111/j.1547-5069.1989.tb00148.x

HITComp. (2017). Health information technology competencies. Retrieved from http://hitcomp.org

Hunt, E. C., Sproat, S. B., & Kitzmiller, R. R. (2004). *The nursing informatics implementation guide.* New York, NY: Springer Publishing.

McGonigle, D., & Mastrian, K. G. (2014). *Nursing informatics and the foundation of knowledge* (3rd ed.). Burlington, MA: Jones & Bartlett Learning.

National Council of State Boards of Nursing. (2017). eNLC implementation. Retrieved from https://www.ncsbn.org/enhanced-nlc-implementation.htm

Ronquillo, C., Currie, L. M., & Rodney, P. (2016). The evolution of data-information-knowledge-wisdom in nursing informatics. *Advances in Nursing Science, 39*(1), E1–E18. doi:10.1097/ANS.0000000000000107

Sensmeier, J. (2012). Informatics nurses: What? Where? And how many? Retrieved from http://www.himss.org/sites/himssorg/files/HIMSSorg/Session1_InformaticsNursesWhatWhereHowMany_JoyceSensmeier.pdf

Sutherland, K. (2013). Applying Lewin's change management theory to the implementation of bar-coded medication administration. *Canadian Journal of Nursing Informatics, 8*(1-2). Retrieved from http://cjni.net/journal/?p=2888

U. S. Department of Health & Human Services. (2015). Methods for de-identification of PHI. Retrieved from https://www.hhs.gov/hipaa/for-professionals/privacy/special-topics/de-identification/index.html#protected

U. S. Department of Health & Human Services. (2017a). Enforcement highlights. Retrieved from https://www.hhs.gov/hipaa/for-professionals/compliance-enforcement/data/enforcement-highlights/index.html

U. S. Department of Health & Human Services. (2017b). The HIPAA privacy rule. Retrieved from https://www.hhs.gov/hipaa/for-professionals/privacy/index.html

U. S. Department of Health & Human Services. (2017c). The security rule. Retrieved from https://www.hhs.gov/hipaa/for-professionals/security/index.html

10

The Role of the Nurse Executive

Bonnie Pierce

OBJECTIVES

1. Explain how the nurse executive (NE) specialty differs from other specialties.
2. Examine theories used as an NE.
3. Describe the legal issues impacting an NE.
4. Apply ethics to the NE role in practice.

THE ROLE OF THE NURSE EXECUTIVE

The role of the NE is complex and easily misunderstood. This chapter addresses significant elements of that complexity with a goal of increasing understanding of this demanding yet infinitely rewarding role. Becoming an NE can be a clearly planned professional objective or can come as a surprise, even to the nurse who becomes one. The following story is about a woman who overcame barrier after barrier to follow her passion in life, and in the process ultimately defined the role of the NE.

She wanted to be a nurse, and the nurse she became revolutionized healthcare (Steele, 2017). She could not get support from her family to receive nursing education, but she persevered and attended two different trainings that were offered at the time (Selanders, 2017). She started working as a nurse, and soon found herself reorganizing her facility and improving outcomes and efficiency. She promoted nurses as leaders in healthcare reform (Nightingale, 1859), and she modeled the behavior.

She understood that women were treated as subordinates and nurses were not viewed as professionals. To overcome these cultural barriers, she knew she would have to demonstrate extraordinary administrative acumen (Steele, 2017). She was mission-driven and a woman of deep faith (Selanders, 2017). She lived her mission, "to serve humankind by promoting wellness and preventing senseless morbidity and mortality" (Steele, 2017, p. 57). When war broke out, she wrote to the Secretary of War, requesting to take nurses to a foreign country to decrease the mortality rate of wounded soldiers. The Secretary of War was of a like mind, and her request was granted (Selanders, 2017). The war was in the Crimea, the nurse was Florence Nightingale, and the year was 1854.

Ms. Nightingale and her nurses were deployed to the hospital in Scutari. On arrival, Ms. Nightingale found that hospital conditions and logistics for acquisition of needed supplies were at best inadequate and at worst deplorable. She immediately set in motion a multifaceted approach to address these deficiencies. Nevertheless, the medical staff was not supportive until the hospital was overwhelmed with incoming wounded (Selanders, 2017). Her theory of nursing emphasized a clean environment, good nutrition, and an orderly and quiet environment that put the patient in the best situation for healing (Steele, 2017). To address the crisis, Ms. Nightingale ordered supplies with money she had been provided, recruited volunteers, especially the wives of soldiers, to do laundry, and organized the nurses to clean the barracks and provide nursing care. She obtained support from England to repair the hospital so that there was clean running water, ventilation, and drainage of sewage (Steele, 2017). She established standards for care, including adequate nutrition, bathing, and clean clothing and bandages. She also addressed the psychosocial needs of the wounded by helping them write letters back home and providing educational activities (Selanders, 2017).

Weeks and months passed. Ms. Nightingale revamped recordkeeping in the Scutari hospital and introduced statistics. She had previously learned how to represent data visually and introduced the polar chart into healthcare, graphing the sharp decline in the mortality rate, from 42.7% to 2.2% (Steele, 2017), since she arrived and implemented the numerous interventions noted earlier. Once the improvement in outcomes was apparent, Ms. Nightingale received the respect of soldiers, medical staff, and the nurses alike. She made rounds, most notably at night using her lamp for light, provided direct patient care, and kept meticulous records. She focused on the environment of care. All of her interventions taken together changed healthcare for the better. Her changes remain important to the healthcare system to this day.

Ms. Nightingale embodied the role of the NE. She refused to accept the status quo, had a guiding theory for nursing care, and implemented it against tremendous odds. She was resilient in the face of crisis and demonstrated the value of nurses and nursing administration to harsh critics and the world at large. She conceptualized a distinct role for nurses, separate from physicians, which focused on promoting health through the concepts of person, health, and environment (Arnone & Fitzsimons, 2015). She professionalized nursing and remains a quintessential exemplar of executive nursing practice.

Now, in the 21st century, The Joint Commission (TJC) defines, and the American Organization of Nurse Executives (AONE) develops competencies for, the role of the NE (AONE, 2015). The role of the NE has expanded in the late 20th and early 21st centuries from solely focusing on the delivery of nursing care to include supervision of numerous disciplines such as social work, chaplaincy, pharmacy, sterile processing, nutrition, and other services that cross the continuum of care (Nurses for a Healthier Tomorrow, 2006). The NE reports to the Chief Executive Officer of the health system. This alignment establishes the position as an executive, with the concomitant responsibility and authority.

As executive leaders, NEs are responsible to acquire and use resources to create an environment that is healthy for nurses and healing for their patients. The NE collaborates with the executive team to design patient care delivery systems. Acting as a role model for nurses, the NE advances the practice of nursing and builds relationships with multiple disciplines across the organization. As a healthcare leader, the NE makes connections and advocates for improved outcomes across the spectrum of healthcare, within the organization and in the broader community (Pierce, 2015). NEs are dual-hatted, with the competency and responsibility to advance clinical care and to establish and manage multimillion-dollar budgets. They promote new ways of thinking to achieve excellence in nursing practice that improve outcomes for patients and the healthcare system (AONE, 2015; Nurses for a Healthier Tomorrow, 2006).

THE ROLE OF THE NURSE EXECUTIVE

Nursing has theories about nursing practice from multiple renowned authors and thinkers. These theories are important to shape and guide nursing practice at the individual and institutional level. The discussion of the depth and breadth of multiple nursing theories is beyond the scope of this chapter, and readers are recommended to look further into the work of theorists such as Patricia Benner, Virginia Henderson, Margaret Newman, Florence Nightingale, Dorothea Orem, Hildegard Peplau, Martha E. Rogers, Sister Callista Roy, and Jean Watson to enrich their understanding of nursing theory. The work of Benner as applicable to nursing practice and the NE is described in the following text.

It is important for the NE to use a theoretical approach to guide nursing practice. The American Nurses Credentialing Center (ANCC) requires that a nursing theory be apparent and in use throughout the hospital to attain their Magnet® and Pathway to Excellence designations. The NE is charged with leading the implementation of the theoretical approach for the facility. The ANCC developed the Magnet Recognition Program to recognize and promote nursing practice settings in which nurses are supported to deliver high-quality care. The three overarching goals of the program are to (a) promote quality of nursing care in settings that support professional nursing practice; (b) identify excellence in nursing care delivery; and (c) disseminate best practices in nursing (ANCC, 2017). Hospitals with Magnet designation indicate to the public that they observe reliable standards by which consumers can expect to receive high-quality care.

The application of theory to the role of the NE is also important. The NE is encouraged to use nursing theory to guide nurses in their practice. However, because the position of NE encompasses both clinical and business practices, the use of theory for this role is ideally expanded to include not only nursing theory but also theory from the business community as well. In this chapter, the use of a developmental theory for the NE that starts with the work of Benner and evolves into the work of William Torbert is articulated. The relevance of a developmental theory for NEs is first explored by examining the Magnet Model.

THE ROLE OF THE NURSE EXECUTIVE TO ACHIEVE MAGNET RECOGNITION

As noted earlier, Magnet organizations demonstrate high nursing standards and patient outcomes. The NE leaders of these organizations are required to work within the executive team to lead the whole facility toward excellence as defined by the Magnet Model. Their ability to accomplish this goal requires an advanced skill set. The role of the NE figures prominently in this model.

The Magnet Model contains five components (ANCC, 2008). The model is a reorganization of the original 14 Forces of Magnet. Each model component contains one or more of the 14 forces. The first model component is transformational leadership (TL). The TL model component includes force number (1), quality of nursing leadership, and number (3), management style.

The ANCC (2008) defines *TL* as "Leadership that identifies and communicates vision and values and asks for the involvement of the work group to achieve the vision" (p. 45). In addition, the ANCC (2008) states the following about new skills required of the TL:

> *The transformational leader must lead people to where they need to be to meet the demands of the future. This requires vision, influence, clinical knowledge, and a strong expertise relating to professional nursing practice. It also acknowledges that transformation may create turbulence and involve atypical approaches to solutions.*

As described in the forces and the model, Magnet facilities require a strong and visionary NE to guide and support excellence in nursing practice that is supported by a professional environment. These leaders and the professional practice they support must not only elevate the standards of the nursing profession but also help their organizations transform to meet patient care and organizational needs in a turbulent healthcare environment. TL is necessary to innovate methods for delivering care that increase efficiency, safety for staff and patients, and accessibility to care. This level of innovation requires enhanced change management practices and strategic thinking.

Structural empowerment is the second of the five Magnet Model components. The visionary leaders develop structures and programs to support empowerment of the staff, including relationships with the community to support the image of nursing and staff development. The mission, vision, values, and the strategic priorities of the organization are achieved through the resulting engagement and empowerment of the staff. The leadership also heavily influences the remaining model components; however, the focus here is on the leadership components of the NE role.

The ANCC lists leading as the first primary domain of the NE (ANCC, 2005). It designed the Magnet recognition process with a detailed focus on the NE as a person, a professional, and a leader. The purpose of the Magnet Recognition Program is to provide a framework to recognize excellence in several areas that also define essential aspects of the role of the NE. The Magnet purpose (and role definition) elements are as follows:

- The management philosophy and practices of nursing services

- Adherence to standards for improving the quality of patient care

- Leadership of the nurse administrator in supporting professional practice and continued competence of nursing personnel

- Attention to the cultural and ethnic diversity of patients and their significant others, as well as the care providers in the system (McClure & Hinshaw, 2002, p. 13)

This list describes everyday responsibilities of the NE role. When the role is optimally implemented, the NE in Magnet organizations establishes the vision and leads with ideas, and the nurse managers move forward with these ideas and work with the staff to implement them (McClure & Hinshaw, 2002).

As described earlier, the role of the NE in the Magnet Recognition Program is central to an organization's success in being recognized as a Magnet. TL is the first component of the Magnet model and is an important leadership style for the NE to master. Marshall (2011) underscores in her text that the ability to be transformational leaders is essential for nurses to lead effectively. The skill set of TL is, however, more than a leadership style. It is an essential aspect of the leader who is able to accomplish enhanced changed management and strategic thinking.

The importance of TL as an essential aspect of the business leader was established by Rooke and Torbert (2005). The highly competent NE and/or business leader would have necessarily undergone extraordinary personal development to incorporate the skill of transformation as a stable aspect of their personalities. Rooke and Torbert (2005) found that only 5% of leaders they worked with developed this transformational capacity. However, the Magnet Model and numerous authors expound upon the importance of TL for NEs. The role of developmental theory then becomes applicable to the NE and the business leader.

Explanation of Developmental Theory

Piaget (1972) studied the development of children from infancy to adolescence, noting predictable stages as a child develops physically and intellectually. Subsequently, other psychologists studied development in children, adolescents, and adults of multiple types of intelligence, moral development, and stages of consciousness (Gardner, 2011; Kohlberg, 1984; Wilber, 2000; Wilber, 2011). Benner (1984) documented the development of the practice of nurses through predictable stages. Developmental theories include all of these attributes for the purpose of explaining and promoting human development (Cook-Greuter, 2004). The distinctive characteristic of developmental theory is that the accomplishments in lower stages of development occur predictably, in a defined order, and are essential precursors for development to higher stages (Loevinger, 1966).

Benner, Tanner, and Chesla (1992) describe nurses' development as they gain experience and ability to respond to contextual cues and patterns. She refers to four levels of developmental expertise in nurses: advanced beginner, competent, proficient, and expert. Each level of nurse sees patients and the clinical environment in a different way. The nurse at each level has a progressively more complex ability to understand and respond to the situation.

Benner et al. (1992) define newly licensed nurses as advanced beginners. They need checklists and organize themselves around tasks and documentation. They learn about clinical situations through experiencing them in real life, not just in theory. Competent nurses, those at the next level of development, still rely heavily on theoretical underpinnings and complex routines. They have begun to see more aspects of clinical situations than the advanced beginner, but are driven by goals and plans rather than context.

The more significant change occurs at the next level of growth within the proficient nurse (Benner et al., 1992). The context of the situation takes priority over plans, and nuances stand out that would have been missed in earlier stages of development. This understanding of the clinical environment demonstrates increased judgment as well as perception, and is accompanied by the nurse experiencing that they are doing more good in their work.

The highest level in Benner's (1984) developmental theory for nurses is the expert nurse. At this level, the nurse expects relevant aspects of the clinical situation to change, takes action on elements that emerge as significant according to her or his perception, and understands the perception that other clinicians have of the situation. This complexity is best revealed in the stories the nurses tell about their experiences in healthcare settings (Benner et al., 1992).

Benner's developmental concepts are readily applied in nursing settings. However, the role of the NE also demands business expertise. Torbert and Cook-Greuter (2004) present a developmental theory that has common themes with Benner's, and their theory has been used to predict who is most likely to be successful in business (Rooke & Torbert, 2005). An explanation of that theory follows.

Action-Logic as a Developmental Theory

Torbert and Cook-Greuter (2004) name the stages in their developmental theory action-logics and describe them further using terms illustrative of each action-logic. Action-logics are "strategies, schemas, ploys, game plans, typical modes of reflecting on experience" (Torbert & Cook-Greuter, 2004, p. 22). When a person inhabits an action-logic, that action-logic is the way he or she experiences the world, his or her worldview. The theory of action-logics explains an important concept for leaders: The ability to create and implement strategy requires a highly developed action-logic.

Leaders demonstrate one of seven action-logics. More action-logics are described, but were not found in leaders in the research presented by Rooke, Torbert, and Cook-Greuter. Each action-logic is a distinct stage of development. The action-logics are grouped into categories named preconventional, conventional, and postconventional (Torbert & Cook-Greuter, 2004). There is only one action-logic in the preconventional stage found in leaders, and it is called Opportunistic. This action-logic is typical in children, and most of them develop beyond this stage during adolescence. The Diplomat, Expert, and Achiever action-logics belong to the conventional category. Persons in conventional action-logics place a high value on stability and seek out similarity. They rely on social and power structures and norms to establish stability. Persons in the postconventional action-logics, Individualists, Strategists, and Alchemists, engage in ongoing creative personal transformation and appreciate change and diversity (Torbert & Cook-Greuter, 2004). The use of action-logics as a developmental tool was concentrated in the business community.

Rooke and Torbert (2005) published research they conducted over 25 years in which they implemented survey-based consulting at numerous for-profit and nonprofit businesses and governmental agencies in America and Europe. They worked with firms that included Deutsche Bank, Harvard Pilgrim Healthcare, Hewlett-Packard, Trillium Asset Management, Aviva, and Volvo. They used their developmental theory to help executives in these companies improve their leadership skills. They assisted thousands of leaders with this process.

Part of the process included the use of a 36-item sentence completion test. The sentences in the profile begin with a phrase such as "A good leader..." (Rooke & Torbert, 2005, p. 68) and the participant completes the sentence. The responses vary, but vary predictably. Highly skilled evaluators interpret the responses, which are then placed into an action-logic profile. The action-logic represents the leader's manner of thinking and responding, especially when challenged or under stress.

Action-Logic as a Predictor of Success

Rooke and Torbert (2005) discovered a correlation between a leader's action-logic and his or her success in business. They learned that business leaders who had only developed conventional action-logics were less successful than business leaders who had achieved postconventional (more highly developed) action-logics. Not only did the higher action-logic correlate with the leaders' personal success but it also correlated with the success of the businesses within which they worked.

Rooke and Torbert (2005) found that the success of businesses was associated with the leaders' ability to transform themselves, and to also transform their company. They observed that below-average performance was associated with leaders displaying action-logics called Opportunist, Diplomat, and Expert. (It is important to note that the definitions for Expert used by Torbert and Benner are different. More discussion to clarify similarities and differences in their theories follows in the section "Comparison Between Benner's and Torbert and Cook-Greuter's Theories.") Additional illustrations of characteristics of the preconventional and conventional level action-logics are given as follows:

1. The opportunist will be self-centered, break rules, and engage in win-lose scenarios, like the leaders of the energy company Enron. This is a preconventional action-logic.

2. A diplomat avoids conflict and tries too hard to be nice and make everything look good. Avoidance of conflict by a senior leader ultimately results in failure. This is a conventional action-logic.

3. An expert thinks he or she knows best, respects only those with very similar knowledge, and will likely drive away numerous senior managers because of his or her failure to collaborate. This is a conventional action-logic.

Once the leaders' action-logics increased to the Achiever level, the outcomes improved. These leaders were able to implement strategies that had a positive impact on the organization. In addition, these leaders had good conflict resolution skills and became positive role models for the employees. They could lead their team to accomplish both short- and long-term goals, decrease staff turnover, and increase business income more than leaders with the Expert action-logic who ran similar businesses. This is also a conventional action-logic. One of the important shortcomings of this action-logic is the lack of the ability to accept disconfirmatory feedback. The leaders can accept only feedback that confirms their own view (Torbert & Cook-Greuter, 2004).

Sustained business success was achieved only by organizations with leaders displaying Individualist, Strategist, or Alchemist action-logics. These are postconventional action-logics. These leaders and their companies were consistently able to transform to become and/or remain successful. Leaders with the Individualist action-logic have enhanced awareness and have a reputation for increasing efficiency and decreasing cost. Leaders who have the Strategist action-logic are able to create a vision that can be shared by people with all action-logics, which becomes compelling to the employees. This engagement then supports personal and corporate transformation. The

Alchemist action-logic is rarely found within corporations and produces outcomes at corporate and societal levels. The Alchemist creates transformation by integrating material and spiritual concerns of the members of the society to transform the culture at important moments in the life of the society.

Comparison Between Benner's and Torbert and Cook-Greuter's Theories

The NE must demonstrate excellence both as a clinician and as a business leader. Benner's theory illustrates the process nurses go through as they develop through the stages she describes. Torbert and Cook-Greuter describe stages that share characteristics with Benner's stages. Benner notes that as nurses gain experience, they see situations differently. Torbert and Cook-Greuter describe each stage as a worldview.

Benner notes that inexperienced nurses rely on rules and seek to establish stability. As nurses advance, they improve in their ability to recognize patterns. This skill eventually helps them let go of heavy emphasis on stability and external theories and increases their reliance on their intuitive grasp of the situation. The Expert nurse, in Benner's theory, no longer relies on stability but anticipates changes and can sense others' grasp of the situation.

Each of these theorists uses Expert to describe a stage, but the use of the term differs between Benner and Torbert and Cook-Greuter. The Expert action-logic describes a person who is similar to the competent nurse in his or her heavy reliance on theory and external routines to gain control. The Expert action-logic is also much more restricted in its awareness of others than Benner's Expert.

Torbert and Cook-Greuter note that leaders with conventional action-logics seek stability and those with postconventional action-logics appreciate transformation instead. The postconventional action-logics embody increasing awareness that radically alters the way those within these stages experience the world. Although it is beyond the scope of this chapter to directly compare Benner's stages with action-logics, it appears that Benner's Expert stage may be a postconventional stage in Torbert and Cook-Greuter's theory.

The Importance of the Theory of Action-Logics for NEs

Benner notes that experience and support are needed for the process of development in nurses to unfold optimally. Torbert and Cook-Greuter describe in detail actions that can be taken to support advancement from one action-logic to the next. Because the need for the ability to design and implement strategy is so important in the healthcare system, it has become critical to use the developmental theory of action-logics to help NEs become the most effective transformational leaders possible.

One must work to advance one's action-logic to use the theory. Although a thorough discussion of the topic is beyond the scope of this chapter, a few concepts are presented to encourage the reader to engage in further exploration. It is important to reiterate that action-logics can be advanced in any person who is capable of abstract thought. Any individual serious about being a good and successful leader can undertake this journey and experience lasting personal and organizational benefits.

It is helpful to know your own action-logic to know which activities and persons to have on your support team that are the most likely to promote your growth. Torbert and Cook-Greuter (2004) discuss action inquiry as a tool to advance action-logic through enhancing awareness, effectiveness, integrity, mutuality, and sustainability in ourselves and in our work. Ideally, action inquiry is conducted in a collaborative rather than in a competitive manner. To begin using action inquiry, Torbert and Cook-Greuter (2004) state, "The first step is to begin to recognize how limited our ordinary attention and awareness is. The second step is to begin exercising our awareness in new ways in the midst of challenging situations" (p. 21). They recommend the practice of noticing how you are feeling multiple times a day. Noticing can be done every hour, or at mealtime and before bed, or as you transition from one activity to another. The exercise is to notice how you are feeling. Also, notice moments during the day that are the least satisfying and the most satisfying. Think about why you experienced these moments as positive or negative.

Next, pay attention to yourself and others in conversation. Pay attention to whether the conversations result in one person influencing primarily or whether all persons in the conversation mutually influence one another. Notice whether you are using all four parts of speech emphasized as important by Torbert and Cook-Greuter (2004), namely, framing, advocating, illustrating, and inquiring. Torbert and Cook-Greuter state that mastering the understanding and use of these methods of speaking will increase one's awareness and effectiveness. The definitions of these terms follow:

Framing refers to explicitly stating what the purpose is for the present occasion, what the dilemma is that everyone is at the meeting to resolve, and what assumptions you think are shared or not shared (but need to be tested out loud to be sure; p. 28).

Advocating refers to explicitly asserting an option, perception, feeling, or strategy for action in relatively abstract terms (p. 28).

Illustrating involves telling a bit of a concrete story that puts meat on the bones of the advocacy and thereby orients and motivates others more clearly (p. 29).

Inquiring involves questioning others to learn something from them (p. 29).

It is important when engaging in action inquiry to encourage people, when you inquire of them, to voice their true opinions. One's assumptions and perceptions must be tested and expanded for one to grow. Also, producing a mutual benefit is a goal for persons with more advanced action logics.

Another helpful practice is to meet monthly with other persons interested in supporting your growth and/or supporting growth in themselves to reflect on each other's experiences. The group would consider how individuals used the four parts of speech in conversations with others, and they would examine how they felt during the interactions. Torbert and Cook-Greuter (2004) suggest additional helpful methods to enhance naming of feelings and increasing one's awareness of how they impact others. Explore their work and the work of their associates for additional information.

This section has discussed the importance of the use of theory by and for NEs. A developmental theory has been described to help NEs be maximally effective and fulfilled. The chapter now discusses the role of the NE as defined by nursing and other healthcare organizations.

ORGANIZATIONAL DESCRIPTIONS OF THE NURSE EXECUTIVE

The role of the NE is described by several nursing professional organizations, by a group of nursing professional organizations in collaboration with other healthcare disciplines, and by TJC. Additionally, the American Nurses Association (2016) has established the scope of and standards of nursing administrative practice. The standards follow the nursing process, and applied at the executive level are: (1) assessment (2); identification of problems, issues and trends (3); outcomes identification (4); planning (5); implementation, including care coordination, health teaching and promotion; and (6) evaluation.

The American Nurses Association through the ANCC (2005) defines the NE as "the nurse who is responsible for organized nursing services and manages from the perspective of the organization as a whole. Her/his five primary domains of activity are leading, collaborating, facilitating, integrating, and evaluating" (p. 33). The ANCC provides national certification for the role of the NE, the Nurse Executive–Board Certified (NE-BC).

The AONE posts a position description for a chief nursing officer (CNO) on their website. The term NE as used in this chapter is synonymous with the term CNO. The position description applies to either a CNO for a system of hospitals or the CNO of one facility. The position summary within that job description follows:

This position has overall accountability for providing leadership, direction, and administration of day-to-day operations associated with direct patient care activities and clinical education and development, including continuous improvement of nursing services and staff to meet the needs and expectations of those served by the System, at assigned facility or campus while maintaining a high level of visibility at the facility, region and system levels. Ensures the realization of quality and economical health care services within facility and system guidelines and philosophies. This position is responsible for driving, supporting and modeling a service-oriented culture focused on employee engagement, quality, patient safety, service excellence, fiscal responsibility, and the overall patient experience. Serves as a member of the executive leadership team at the facility and system levels, building and supporting effective collegial relationships with applicable internal and external constituents and stakeholders and ensuring optimal operating effectiveness and strategic positioning. (AONE, 2017, para. 1)

This statement is an introductory summary; additional elements of the role are included in the job description. Education required is a bachelor of science in nursing with a master's in a related field. A minimum of 7 to 10 years of progressively responsible nursing leadership positions and a current license as a registered nurse are also required. The ability to handle multiple responsibilities, work with executives across the system, pay attention to detail, maintain good relationships with schools of nursing, and an interest in lifelong learning are essential aspects of the role. A leadership style that promotes teamwork and thorough communication is necessary. The AONE also provides national certification for the role of the NE, the Certification in Executive Nursing Practice (CENP).

Nurses for a Healthier Tomorrow is a coalition of 43 professional nursing and healthcare organizations that work together to promote nursing and attract people into the profession (Nurses for a Healthier Tomorrow, 2006). They describe the NE as a leader who acts as a role model to exemplify the mission and vision of his or her organization, values diversity, demonstrates cultural competence in interactions with patients and staff, and supports a patient care environment for staff to do the same. The NE ensures staff receive the education needed to remain competent as techniques change, and provides opportunities for staff to grow and develop in the many areas nurses may work. The NE promotes quality improvement through systems thinking, stays current within the field of NE practice, is effective as both a team member and a team leader, and is fiscally accountable (Nurses for a Healthier Tomorrow, 2006). The role of the nurse in executive practice has evolved from a focus on nursing services to one that is accountable for patient care in multiple disciplines across the continuum of care. The NE reports directly to the CEO of the healthcare organization.

The AONE uses a model for leadership competency that was developed by the Healthcare Leadership Alliance in 2004. In addition to the AONE, other members of the alliance include the American College of Healthcare Executives, the American Association for Physician Leadership, Healthcare Financial Management Association, Healthcare Information and Management Systems Society, and Medical Group Management Association. The relevance of the model is maintained through periodic job analysis studies in which the reliability and validity model domains are evaluated. The most recent study was released in 2014. The model includes the following domains:

- Communication and relationship building

- Knowledge of the healthcare environment

- Leadership

- Professionalism

- Business skills and principles (AONE, 2015, p. 3)

The alliance is developing a common set of leadership competencies for additional healthcare executive roles.

Through the NE competency model, the AONE (2015) has articulated competencies that are important for nursing leaders in each of the domains noted earlier. Several of the examples are as follows:

- "Assert views in non-threatening, non-judgmental ways" (p. 4).

- "Address and model appropriate conflict resolution" (p. 5).

- "Represent patient care issues to the governing body" (p. 6).

- "Discuss, resolve and learn from ethical dilemmas" (p. 9).

The entire document is available online at the website given in AONE (2015). In keeping with the competency, the NE must learn from ethical dilemmas. The section "Ethical Dilemma Case Study" presents a scenario that presents several ethical dilemmas for discussion and resolution.

ETHICAL DILEMMA CASE STUDY

The following case study is an adaptation and amalgamation of stories that have presented themselves at various times during 40 years of professional nursing practice.

The Scenario

Nurse A came in for the night shift. She noticed that her patient, Mr. B, had deteriorating vital signs. She called the doctor on call (Dr. C) for the patient. The doctor failed to respond. After multiple attempts, Nurse A still failed to reach the on-call doctor but reached the Medical Officer of the Day (MOD). She asked the MOD to please come and see the patient, but he refused. She pressed the MOD again and stated she thought an in-person evaluation was needed. The MOD responded, "Where did you get your medical degree?" and refused to see the patient. The nurse shut down emotionally and stopped advocating for the patient. In the morning when the day-shift nurse (Nurse E) came on, she called a rapid response and the patient was transferred to the ICU. The delay in transferring the patient to the ICU resulted in the patient requiring extensive interventions to become stable. The patient had an increased length of stay in the ICU than would have been required had the intensive care he needed not been delayed for almost 12 hours. In truth, however, the patient recovered from the incident more quickly than did Nurse A.

Nurse A came to the NE after this incident to ask for help. She felt she had failed the patient, was angry with the doctors, and still felt powerless to advocate for other patients. She wanted the situation "fixed," including "putting those doctors in their place." The NE now has a responsibility to analyze the situation from an ethical perspective and improve patient safety and psychological safety for the staff.

Scenario Analysis in Ethical Terms

Immanuel Kant describes the ethics of duty, which includes the importance of respecting oneself and other people (Hinman, 2008). Kant writes that two conditions are required for an act to be morally good. First, if an action is done for the sake of duty, the action has moral worth. Second, if the reason behind the action is a universal law, the action is morally correct (Hinman, 2008). A third premise from Kant is that human beings should be treated with respect, including that each person should respect oneself. People should never be treated as a means to an end (Hinman, 2008).

The prima facie (at first glance) evidence appears to show that Nurse A has performed her duty by assessing Mr. B and calling Dr. C. It appears that Dr. C is neglecting his duty as the on-call physician. It appears that the MOD is neglecting his duty by not responding to Nurse A's requests to see the patient. In addition, the MOD mocks Nurse A. Up to this point, it appears that Nurse A is on the moral high ground and the physicians are failing to behave morally because they are not fulfilling their duties, which include treating Nurse A with respect. Their actions are immoral because they have an actual duty to care for Mr. B and treat Nurse A with respect according to what we know of their positions in the agency in this scenario.

Nurse A's emotional response to the lack of responsiveness by the physicians, compounded by being disrespected by being mocked, eventually results in her, too, neglecting her duty. Nurse E performs her duty and ensures the patient receives the care he needs. The apparent ease with which Nurse E accomplishes her duty adds to Nurse A's feelings of frustration.

The NE with a mature action-logic does not rush to judgment. Although it appears that the physicians have obviously shirked their moral obligations, additional analysis is required. The NE can look further into Kant's reasoning concerning self-interest. Kant postulates that performing a duty out of self-interest, rather than out of a pure sense of duty, falls short of being morally worthy.

The NE needs to explore more of the specifics within the scenario. Was Dr. C actually on call? If that is indeed the case and Dr. C still failed to respond, the failure should be reported in writing to Dr. C's supervisor. It is important to confirm the accuracy of the call list the nurse used and ensure nurses always have an accurate on-call list. Nurse A also needs to be transparent about the list she used, even if she might have made the mistake herself about whom to call.

What did Nurse A report to the MOD? Did the MOD have the responsibility for all of the patients in the house? If so, did the nurse give the MOD a clear and complete picture of the patient's condition and how it had changed and over what period of time? If the answer to these questions is yes, then a report in writing should be sent immediately to the MOD's supervisor. However, if the MOD was not organizationally responsible for this patient, or if the nurse gave only a vague or partial report, the MOD may have justification for not seeing the patient. However, the MOD is not justified in mocking Nurse A, and that action should be reported in writing.

The NE needs to evaluate whether, in self-interest, Nurse A is reporting the incidents to retaliate and to cover up for errors she may have made. A lesson learned could be to ensure that Nurse A understands the importance of giving a thorough report to the provider. A thorough report provides a complete description of the patient, including vital signs, skin assessment, heart, lung, and abdominal assessment, the change in status over a defined period of time, and any additional information pertinent to the patient. Giving this level of assessment to the provider assists the provider in giving an informed response that will address the patient's needs.

Nurse A needs to understand the organization sufficiently to know who to call for help. If the MOD is supposed to respond and does not, who does the nurse call next? Everyone has a boss, and the NE must ensure that all nurses know how to call up the chain of command to get assistance for their patients. A list of the physicians' chain of command is needed with phone numbers so nurses can call for help. Calling up the chain can also include calling the Nursing Officer of the Day, or the nurse's immediate supervisor, or even the NE for assistance. The staff nurse must have access to these numbers. An alternative to calling up the physician or nursing chain of command is to call a rapid response. The most important thing is for Nurse A and all nursing staff to have options that they can exercise quickly to get the care their patients need. The NE needs to ensure all staff feel encouraged and supported to make these calls.

Ideally, the NE will enlist Nurse A to assist in teaching her peers whom or what to call when the initial attempts do not produce the needed results. The NE also will need to discuss with the executive leadership the effect that disrespect in the workplace has on the psychological safety of the staff and ultimately on the care of the patient. The entire team will need to put in place personal, social, and structural supports for speaking up across the organization (Maxfield, Grenny, Ramón, & Groah, 2011) to help all staff speak up for patient safety.

Speaking Up as a Challenging But Ethical Imperative

Maxfield et al. (2011) found that 58% of a group of 2,383 nurses had experiences in which an unsafe situation had developed, and they felt "unsafe to speak up or were unable to get others to listen" (p. 2). At first blush, it is easy to think that these nurses are just lacking the moral courage to speak up. However, Maxfield et al. (2011) demonstrate that multiple elements must be in place to overcome what they found to be a culture of organizational silence that prevents the majority of nurses from speaking up. Staff must develop personal skill in speaking up. The personal skill must be supported socially by their peers and especially by the physician staff. The organization's leaders must reward speaking up and extinguish the barriers to speaking up. Maxfield et al. (2011) articulate barriers to speaking up and define supports to help eliminate those barriers.

Pierce (2015) explored the barriers and the supports for speaking up used by NEs of Magnet facilities in the Veterans Health Administration. Pierce (2015) found that a postconventional action-logic assisted the NE to provide more supports for speaking up than a conventional action-logic. Pierce (2015) also found that persistence pays in overcoming barriers to speaking up. In the stories told by the Magnet NEs, speaking up once about a problem never successfully addressed the issue. At least two speaking-up interventions were always required to overcome one barrier to speaking up. In all but one instance, it required more than a 2:1 ratio of speaking-up behaviors to barriers encountered to address the issue. The ratio of speaking-up efforts to barriers was 9:1 in one situation before the NE was able to arrive at a sustained resolution to the problem. NEs and nursing staff need to know that speaking up requires multiple iterations to achieve the outcomes desired and the outcomes that patients need.

NEs must be able to provide psychologically safe environments so nurses will be able to speak up. NEs must develop their own leadership maturity so they can enhance their ability to support nurses speaking up and to accurately hear what the nurses have to say. The NEs who possess a conventional action-logic embody a significant barrier to speaking up: They do not listen deeply, and they discount information that does not conform to their worldview. They are completely unaware of this limitation because it is a function of a conventional action-logic. Their inability to fully support speaking up and to listen fully is certainly not intentional, because they will tell you that speaking up is a moral imperative and they support it. However, their skills and ability to support speaking up personally and to get the executive team to support speaking up are hampered by their action-logic. Once they advance their action-logic to the postconventional stages, their ability to support speaking up personally and organizationally takes a significant leap forward. Therefore, it becomes a moral imperative for NEs to develop their leadership maturity into the postconventional action-logics. Their staff and their patients need the NE to embody this level of development to improve the healthcare system.

The challenge to enhance leadership maturity in the NE brings this chapter full circle. The developmental theories of Benner and Torbert help the NE to grow as a nurse, as a business leader, and as a person. This growth is an ethical imperative so the NE can be the ethical leader who fulfills the duty of supporting speaking up for nurses. Nursing started with a postconventional thinker in Ms. Nightingale. She changed healthcare for the better and for all time. I hope that current and future NEs will rise to the challenge of continuing their growth in leadership maturity, for they, too, will potentially impact healthcare for generations to come.

CRITICAL THINKING QUESTIONS

1. Discuss the similarities and differences between a clinical nurse leader and an NE.

2. What differences do you see between developmental theory and action logic?

3. How could you use action logic in your current role?

4. Present a time where you may have felt unable to fully advocate for a patient. Did you feel supported by an NE? How so? If not, how would that support have made a difference?

REFERENCES

American Nurses Association. (2016). *Nursing administration: Scope and standards of practice*. Siver Spring, MD: Author.

American Nurses Credentialing Center. (2005). *The Magnet Recognition Program application manual*. Silver Spring, MD: Author.

American Nurses Credentialing Center. (2008). *The Magnet Model components and sources of evidence*. Silver Spring, MD: Author.

American Nurses Credentialing Center. (2017). Magnet program overview. Retrieved from http://www.nursecredentialing.org/Magnet/ProgramOverview

American Organization of Nurse Executives. (2015). AONE nurse executive competencies. Retrieved from http://www.aone.org/resources/nurse-leader-competencies.shtml

American Organization of Nurse Executives. (2017). Job descriptions. *CNO: ALL/Health System*. Retrieved from http://www.aone.org/resources/job-descriptions.shtml

Arnone, J. M., & Fitzsimons, V. (2015). Plato, nightingale, and nursing: Can you hear me now? *International Journal of Nursing Knowledge, 26*(4), 156–162. doi:10.1111/2047-3095.12059

Benner, P. (1984). *From novice to expert: Excellence and power in clinical nursing practice*. Menlo Park, CA: Addison-Wesley.

Benner, P., Tanner, C., & Chesla, C. (1992). From beginner to expert: Gaining a differentiated clinical world in critical care nursing. *Advances in Nursing Science*, *14*(3), 13–28. doi:10.1097/00012272-199203000-00005

Cook-Greuter, S. R. (2004). Making the case for a developmental perspective. *Industrial and Commercial Training*, *36*(7), 275–281. doi:10.1108/00197850410563902

Gardner, H. (2011). *Frames of mind: The theory of multiple intelligences*. New York, NY: Basic Books.

Hinman, L. M. (2008). *Ethics: A pluralistic approach to moral theory* (4th ed.). Belmont, CA: Thomson/Wadsworth.

Kohlberg, L. (1984). *The psychology of moral development: The nature and validity of moral stages* (Vol. 2). San Francisco, CA: Harper & Row.

Loevinger, J. (1966). The meaning and measurement of ego development. *American Psychologist*, *21*(3), 195–206. doi:10.1037/h0023376

Marshall, E. S. (2011). *Transformational leadership in nursing: From expert clinician to influential leader*. New York, NY: Springer Publishing.

Maxfield, D., Grenny, J., Ramón, L., & Groah, L. (2011). The silent treatment: Why safety tools and checklists aren't enough to save lives. Retrieved from https://www.psqh.com/analysis/the-silent-treatment-why-safety-tools-and-checklists-arent-enough/

McClure, M. L., & Hinshaw, A. S. (Eds.). (2002). *Magnet hospitals revisited: Attraction and retention of professional nurses*. Silver Spring, MD: American Nurses Association.

Nightingale, F. (1859). *Notes on nursing: What it is and what it is not*. London, UK: Harrison & Sons.

Nurses for a Healthier Tomorrow. (2006, April 4). Nurse executive. Retrieved from http://www.nursesource.org/executive.html

Piaget, J. (1972). Intellectual evolution from adolescence to adulthood. *Human Development*, *15*, 1–12. doi:10.1159/000271225

Pierce, B. R. (2015). *Action-logics of Veterans Health Administration Magnet nurse executives and their practice of supporting nurses to speak up* (Doctoral dissertation). Retrieved from https://pqdtopen.proquest.com/doc/1752116799.html?FMT=ABS

Rooke, D., & Torbert, W. R. (2005). 7 Transformations of Leadership. *Harvard Business Review*, *83*(4), 66–66. Retrieved from https://hbr.org/2005/04/seven-transformations-of-leadership

Selanders, L. (2017). *Florence Nightingale*. Encyclopædia Britannica. Retrieved from https://www.britannica.com/biography/Florence-Nightingale

Steele, N. M. (2017). A time to celebrate: Florence Nightingale. *Urologic Nursing*, *37*(2), 57–59. doi:10.7257/1053-816X.2017.37.2.57

The Joint Commission. (2017). Comprehensive accreditation manual. Retrieved from https://www.jcrinc.com/e-dition-old/

Torbert, W. R., & Cook-Greuter, S. R. (2004). *Action inquiry: The secret of timely and transforming leadership*. San Francisco, CA: Berrett-Koehler.

Wilber, K. (2000). *A brief history of everything* (2nd Rev. ed.). Boston, MA: Shambhala.

Wilber, K. (2011). *Integral psychology: Consciousness, spirit, psychology, therapy*. Boston, MA: Shambhala.

SECTION IV

Role Transition

In Section IV, we dig deeper into the expectations of a master's-prepared nurse. As you know, with more knowledge there are more opportunities and expectations. You may already know what you plan to do with a master's degree and have an idea of what these additional expectations will be. However, you may primarily be thinking about a different job or a promotion within your organization. In the next couple of chapters, some specific expectations of master's-prepared nurses as well as differences between BSN- and MSN-prepared nurses as identified by the American Association of Colleges of Nursing are discussed.

11

MSN as Change Agent

Brenda Scott and Mindy Thompson

OBJECTIVES

1. Identify strategies for change.
2. Explore change theories.
3. Evaluate the role of the MSN-prepared nurse in the change process.
4. Identify key steps of the evidence-based practice process.
5. Evaluate evidence-based practice models for use.

Have you ever heard someone say, "That is the way we have always done it?" This phrase is highly frustrating. To me, this attitude shows a lack of growth, an acceptance of circumstance, arrogance, complacency, and fear of change or innovation. As you are aware, healthcare changes rapidly. This change includes roles, processes, and all aspects of the healthcare industry. According to the American Association of Colleges of Nursing (AACN) MSN Essentials (2011), one key aspect of the MSN-prepared nursing role is that of a change leader.

THE ROLE OF THE MSN IN CHANGE

All nurses are leaders, regardless of their position, through their advocating, teaching, and empowering. However, being a change agent often takes a more deliberate approach. Nurses make up the largest portion of the healthcare workforce. With that volume of people, the capability for a collective voice to make a difference could become quite powerful. This is one reason why becoming active members of professional organizations is so important.

You considered an issue or problem and then worked through a process to write up or present a proposal to improve that problem. You provided background information, evidence on why the intervention or solution you proposed should work, cost–benefit analysis, an implementation plan, and an evaluation plan. Now, you may or may not have recognized that the process was and is strikingly similar to the nursing process! You assess the environment or situation, you diagnose a problem, you develop a plan, you find interventions through evidence, you implement those interventions, and then you evaluate the outcomes. See? Nursing process!

So, being a change agent is really just a nursing care plan with some slightly different information. As a nurse, you are constantly assessing. What you may or may not have developed at this point in your career is the process of taking those daily annoyances and/or problems and exploring possible solutions. There are two very important skills in this process that take some practice.

The first of these two skills that are slightly different than that of simple nursing process is identification of stakeholders. We must include every person or group that has a vested interest in the outcome. For instance, if you are trying to solve a patient care issue within a healthcare system, obvious stakeholders are the patients the particular problem impacts and the nurses who take care of those patients. However, there are several others that need to be considered. We work in interdisciplinary environments, and a few questions to help identify additional stakeholders are: What other disciplines would be interested in contributing to the solution? What disciplines do you need support from to make the change successful? Perhaps you need information or action from respiratory therapists, allied health professionals, case managers, or even dietary staff. Another stakeholder you may or may not readily consider is the patient family or caregivers. What is their stake? Of course, they care about the outcome of the patient, but they also greatly contribute to that outcome. One stakeholder we can often forget is administration of the organization where we are trying to make the change. However, they are usually always a key stakeholder. Administration is where money flows to and from. This is the stakeholder that really needs to see and understand your cost–benefit analysis.

When we take care of patients, we tend to focus primarily on that patient or patient group. We must always remember that healthcare is a business, and to provide care to the most people possible, we have to be good stewards of resources that can sometimes be scarce. Sometimes it helps to think of cost–benefit analysis along the lines of benefit versus burden. In healthcare, when you choose one intervention over another, you should weigh the benefit the patient will experience to the burden or complications he or she may experience in the process. Physicians choosing which medication to prescribe is one classic example of benefit versus burden. If a medication is going to cause more side effects than symptoms it will relieve, it may not be a good treatment option. So, relating this back to cost–benefit analysis, your cost is the burden and your benefit is exactly that and numbers are used to illustrate those two categories.

For example, if you are trying to implement a care coordination model to decrease rehospitalization of congestive heart failure patients, you would want to consider how much it costs the hospital when a patient is hospitalized within a certain time frame. You could also consider costs to the patient and family depending on the ultimate goal and outcome you are working toward. By decreasing the rehospitalizations and saving the organization money, you are creating a financial benefit. You also create benefits to the patient, family, nurses, and so forth. See how all of those stakeholders play an important role in change? So, the burden is the cost that it will take to implement the model. Are you hiring new staff? What training will they need? How much will they be paid? What physical space will they need to function? What office equipment will they need? These are all costs that will need to be incurred. Sometimes there is not an immediate financial benefit, so you need to project in a measurable and realistic method to anticipate how long it would take to become beneficial. There are many considerations to cost–benefit analysis and these are closely related and can be guided by whom you identified as a stakeholder.

Once you have decided a change needs to be made and planned what needs to be done, a process to complete this change needs to be used. The process in which change is introduced will often determine whether it is successful. Determining whether an implemented change was successful can be somewhat relative to the assessor. However, there is a pretty good chance you will encounter some resistance to the change you try to implement. As you may have experienced, people may not get overly excited about changes to their routine. Choosing a change theory that will guide you through the process will greatly increase the likelihood of the change taking hold long term.

CHANGE THEORY

Although not a new field of study, change management has seen an incredible growth over the past decade. Change management can be a specialty on its own, but has implications on many other fields including nursing.

Although there are many change theories, nearly all are based on the work of Kurt Lewin, who is often regarded as the father of change management. In this section, we review several theories including Lewin's Change Theory, Spradley's Change Theory, and the Shewhart's cycle. As you may be aware, these are not all the theories of change and are not designed to influence or advocate for any theory above another.

Lewin's Change Theory

In 1947, Lewin introduced the world to his theory on change that is often called changing as three steps (CATS; Lewin, 1947). This theory is frequently used and found throughout nursing, nursing education, and nursing research. In his theory, Lewin described three stages: unfreezing, freezing, and refreezing. Lewin's theory described forces that he labeled as driving, resisting, and equilibrium. In his theory, the driving forces are the leaders and individuals who are pushing change in the organization. As you can probably imagine, the resistant forces are those who do not want the change and are standing in the way of the change implementation. Equilibrium occurs when the resistant and driving balances are equal and no change occurs. These three forces all play an important role in each of the three stages.

Unfreezing

The unfreezing stage is somewhat of a compromise and requires problem solving. In this stage, the object is to reduce the amount of resistance to change., something especially difficult when an organization has been doing the same thing for a long time, has become comfortable, or is opposed to change. Resistance to change does not mean an organization or individual is doing something wrong. Oftentimes, individuals have to be shown why change is necessary. As we discuss in Chapter 13, it is much easier to obtain buy-in with a well-developed communications strategy focused on the why. When the purpose is well communicated to all parties you are attempting to obtain buy-in from, it is easier to move toward unfreezing. As buy-in is obtained or the individuals who resist change are reduced, change can occur. This stage is all about winning the hearts and minds of the people.

Change

In the change stage, a new practice or method of doing things is introduced and implemented. One of the mistakes that many organizations make when implementing change is that they do not have a well-designed plan that allows for the appropriate time to introduce the change. By allowing time to process the change, individuals can go through a process similar to the stages of grief and ultimately make their own decision. This progression allows the individuals to process the change, review the change, and then decide whether they can accept the change. If not, the individuals can make the best decisions for themselves as to their involvement with the project or organization. Once an individual has bought in, accepts, and begins performing the change, the next step is to make it a habit and freeze the behavior.

Freezing

In the freezing stage, the goal is to move from a new change or practice, way of doing things, and eventually replace the old practice with the new. Simply put, the goal is to create a habit. Have you ever heard the old saying that it takes 21 days to create a habit? Science has shown us that old saying is completely false. Lally, van Jaarsveld, Potts, and Wardle (2010) conducted a study of 96 participants who volunteered to develop a new habit. During the 12-week study, observations were collected and on the average it took over 60 days for a habit to develop. After the study, data analysis was conducted and it was determined it would take anywhere from under 20 days to more than 250 to develop a habit (2010). The point here is that habits take time and do not occur immediately. When there is resistance, time needed can increase even more.

One of the biggest challenges of freezing is changing culture. Oftentimes, people throw around the word culture and do not understand what it takes to create a culture or sustain it, let alone change it. Without a culture change, people revert back to previous actions and ways of doing business.

Spradley's Change Theory

Another popular change theory in nursing is Spradley's Change Theory, developed by Barbara Walton Spradley (Longo, 2013). This change theory is similar to the nursing process in that it is made up of assessment, diagnosis, planning, implementation, and evaluation (ADPIE) and shares many similar concepts.

Recognize the Symptoms

The first step of Spradley's change theory is to recognize the symptoms. To be effective, the change agent must be in tune with his or her organization and able to see the signs that a problem exists. Sometimes this recognition is one of the hardest things for a change agent or potential change agent. Although many individuals may choose to ignore the issues or symptoms, a change agent cannot do this and be successful.

Think about patient care; you would not medicate without identifying the symptoms first. As a change agent, you must identify what the symptoms are before you can plan a change. Maybe some of your symptoms include declining patient outcomes, multiple nurse call-ins per shift, or increased supply cost. You must start by identifying these symptoms before moving to the next step in the change process.

Diagnose the Problem

Once a problem has been recognized, the next step is to diagnose the problem. In this step, the change agent will gather and analyze data to determine what is occurring. As with any disease or medical problem, there are usually signs and symptoms, just as with an organization needing change. The change agent may use personal observation, interviews with those who are impacted by the problem, evidence-based practice, industry standards, and many other resources to help determine there is a problem. Once the problem has been identified, data that demonstrate and support the problem can be developed, researched, and refined to support the problem. This problem identification is similar to writing a problem, intervention, comparison, outcome, and time (PICOT) statement in nursing.

Let's see how this process actually may work. If your symptom identification reveals a high turnover rate, as a change agent you will need to dig in to diagnose the problem. After interviews, you identify the problem is with patient ratios. Nurses are leaving your organization because they are required to provide care to too many patients on a given shift. You have reviewed the symptoms and diagnosed the problem. You are now ready to move to the next step in the theory.

Identify Alternative Solutions

The third step is to come up with solutions. In this step, the goal is to identify potential solutions as well as the resources needed to carry out the potential solution. It is also important to know what challenges or roadblocks might keep a solution from being successful in meeting the outcomes of the identified problem. In this step, the change agent will meet with potential stakeholders and look at available solutions. For each proposed solution, the change agent should have an idea of the resources needed, probable budget, potential obstacles, and possible outcomes for each potential solution and have it outlined for all to see.

Let's see the application by considering the same situation presented earlier. You are the nurse leader of the organization where you are experiencing high turnover rates. You have identified that patient-to-nurse ratios are the cause of this turnover. In this phase of the theory, you will need to brainstorm solutions. You may review research to determine best practices, you may review national agencies for recommendations, or you might conduct interviews of those involved to determine what they feel is a reasonable patient-to-nurse ratio. You have identified three potential solutions: hire more unlicensed providers (UPs) to assist the nurses, hire more nurses, and change staffing patterns to decrease the patient-to-nurse ratio from 10:1 to 5:1. You are now ready to move to the next step.

Select Solutions

Once all of the alternatives have been presented, it is up to the change agent or stakeholders to select the solution that solves the problem most completely and is most feasible to execute. During this step, it is sometimes hard to identify what the right solution is. Sometimes the best solution may not be a feasible solution. If a solution takes an excessive amount of money, time, or resources, it is going to be a challenge to get buy-in and acceptance. If the proposed change may be executed in phases, it is important to consider how that might impact your selection of the potential solution. Small steps toward a big outcome can be more helpful than doing nothing.

Let's reconsider our scenario regarding nursing turnover. Although the best solution may be to hire more nurses, hire more UPs, and decrease patient-to-nurse ratios, it may not be realistic for the facility. Let's say this plan would be an additional $2 million required from the budget. Can you see your chief financial officer (CFO) panicking? Most facilities do not have this amount of funds in excess. This type of need would require preplanning and budgeting. You would not be able to decrease patient-to-nurse ratios without hiring.

As the leader of the change, it is your responsibility to develop a thorough plan for review. Consider your current staffing patterns and budget. Is it possible you have a staffing excess on night shift that can be adjusted to cover day shift or vice versa? On reviewing your current staffing, you discover you have 15 nurses working day shift, but only 5 on night shift. You determine that your need on day shift is only 10 nurses. You could develop a plan to move these five extra nurses to night shift to balance staffing. You may also have a hiring plan in place that allows you to hire 15 additional nurses during the next 6 months. Consider hiring the total 15 now with a plan not to hire for the remaining 6 months. You may also determine that you are able to hire two UPs in place of every nurse and still save money. You could consider altering the staffing to incorporate more UPs instead of only hiring nurses. You have several options that can lead to resolving the issue. It will be up to the change agent to determine the next steps.

Plan the Change

Once a change agent has selected a solution, the next step is to plan the change. You may have heard the statement "prior planning prevents poor performance" (there are several variations of this statement ranging from 6 to 12 "P"s depending on the person and their creativity). This adage applies to change management as well. In this step, a proposed change moves from theoretical to actual. Using the solution selected earlier, a detailed action plan to implement the change should be constructed. This action plan should include objectives, benchmarks, and a timeline that is specific, measurable, achievable, realistic, and timely (SMART). The plan must also include a budget that provides the overall cost of the change as well as the cost of sustaining the change and a process of evaluating success. Without identifying what success looks like, it is hard to know when success has been reached and whether the change is positive or needs to be reevaluated. Remember, planning change can be a fluid process.

Let's say you have decided to shuffle a few of your day-shift nurses over to cover the night-shift needs. Your plan will need to include a detailed description of how coverage will improve. You will need to determine how you plan to evaluate the change. Will you plan to implement other strategies at a later point? Will you survey your staff? Will you monitor turnover rate and exit interviews to determine whether this change specifically changed the outcome? These are just a few questions to consider about the plan and evaluation piece. Think about bedside nursing; we do not give a pain medication without evaluation to determine effectiveness. This is the same for change. You cannot implement a solution and never evaluate the results. Healthcare is a data-driven industry and it is important to evaluate effectiveness of change.

Implement the Change

In the implementation phase, the solution is executed using the plan developed in the previous step. In this step, the change agent should use the budget and developed plan to meet the timelines and benchmarks established earlier. This step often includes training, testing, and lots of communication. In many situations, the change agent may not be involved fully in the step. Commonly, other departments within an organization may measure effectiveness or implement the change.

Evaluate the Change

This phase is where the real fun starts. As a change agent, you want to make sure that you have an adequate amount of time to implement a change. Occasionally, it is hard to admit that an idea has not worked as well as you had planned. Think about the nursing process. When an intervention does not work, you do not walk away and stop taking care of the patient. Instead, you consider why an intervention did not work, what to do differently, what data show, and how to move forward. Although informal evaluation occurs throughout the life of the project, formal evaluation is conducted in this phase.

In our scenario, you have reshuffled the staffing patterns to provide more coverage on the night shift. What do you do if your turnover rate increases? This increase could be caused from a number of things. Let's say those day-shift nurses you moved to the night shift could not work that schedule. They chose to leave the unit; this causes turnover rates to increase. Although your solution or change is not failing, you now have another issue to address. In the evaluation period, you may need to readjust the solution as you go. The key is not to give up on addressing the symptoms. This example goes back to patient care; you would not stop providing care if the pain medication you gave 45 minutes ago was ineffective. No, you would provide another solution.

Stabilize the Change

When you achieve the outcomes you want, you have reached this phase. Once evaluation reveals the symptoms have resolved, you can stabilize the change. During this phase, you will make whatever solution you were trying a permanent part of the process. If you arrive at this point, you no longer need to make adjustments. Now, that is not saying you will never make adjustments. If we said that, we would be back to the "way we have always done it" mentality. This step just means that for now the solution works to achieve the outcome expected.

Consider patient care here. You have a patient reporting pain; you give him or her acetaminophen and it resolves the pain. You do not need to give him or her anything else and next time he or she has the same pain, you may try acetaminophen first. When acetaminophen no longer works to resolve the pain, you would need to restart from the first step in this theory.

Shewhart's Cycle

The third change theory we review is Shewhart's cycle. In the 1950s, W. Edward Deming introduced the Shewhart's cycle to the world to revolutionize quality control. This cycle built upon the work of his mentor, grandfather of total quality management, physicist, and statistician Walter Shewhart (Best & Neuhauser, 2006). This cycle was introduced to the Japanese who named it the Deming Circle and Deming Wheel (Moen & Norman, 2010). Commonly, this theory is now referred to as the PDSA cycle: plan, do, study, and act.

Plan

Planning is the first step in the PDSA cycle. It is the most comprehensive step for most change activities. In this step, the change agent will determine the problem, engage with stakeholders, consider possible solutions, and create a plan. You may be thinking, wow that is a lot in one step, and it is certainly. Generally, change does not occur with one person. The change agent typically sees a need and then develops a group of stakeholders to work through the process. This group development is part of this step.

Let's look at this step in action by using the scenario we have considered earlier: high turnover rates. You are the director responsible for a medical–surgical unit and you notice your turnover rates have been drastically increasing. You develop a task force to address this concern. Your task force includes a member of the human resources department, the nurse manager, four charge nurses, and a member of the quality improvement team.

During the "plan" phase, you work with the task force to hold meetings to determine possible solutions. The group agrees on solutions to implement to address the concern. Once the group agrees upon a solution or solutions, you develop a thorough implementation plan. This plan will include budgetary needs, resources, timelines, evaluation criteria, and so forth and will take you to the next step of the cycle.

Do

This step in the cycle is where you implement your selected solution. You may have several solutions that you implement at once or you may have just one. It is important to have a clear plan developed for your implementation process. You will use the plan created during the "plan" phase to guide the "do" phase. At this point, you are merely going to work.

Study

For all you data lovers, this is the step for you. Here you evaluate the solutions to determine whether the outcomes are improving. Any benchmarks and timelines created by the stakeholder group will be used during this cycle. It is very important to determine evaluation criteria during the "plan" phase. If you have not defined what success looks like, you will not know whether your solution should become permanent.

Act

In this phase, you will either solidify the solution as a part of the process or revise and restart the process. No matter how perfect you think a solution will be, sometimes it just does not work. It is important to be flexible in this phase. It is important to review the data generated in the "study" phase. Decisions to move forward with making the change permanent or revising should be based on of the data provided. During this phase, it is important to discuss timelines for review. If you move forward with making a change permanent, it is important to set a goal for a review. You may see this review occurring in 2 years, but this does not mean if another issue arises the change will not be reviewed sooner. If you determine the solution did not impact the outcomes as expected, you would restart with the "plan" phase. If you can visualize a circle, this process is very circular in nature, indicating there is no end to the change process.

EVIDENCE-BASED PRACTICE CHANGE

There are several evidence-based practice models available in the literature. At the core are five basic steps that we cover first. Then we take a look at some variations and discuss some pros and cons.

The Core Process

Strauss (2005) identified five steps in evidence-based practice. These are pretty straightforward in explanation. First and foremost, you need to ask a question. You know you are looking for information about a subject but you need to develop a question you can answer (Strauss, 2005). A PICOT question will come in handy here because it is a format that helps you define a researchable question (Melnyk, 2005). The P in the formula stands for either problem or population depending on what you ask. The I stands for intervention. What is the fix or solution you are trying to apply to the problem or population? C stands for comparison. Comparing two groups, situations, or outcomes will help you define outcome criteria. For example, a PICOT question may be the following: For graduate nursing students (P), will providing explanation of evidence-based practice models (I) versus letting them figure it out on their own (C) help them choose a model that works for them (O) by the end of this chapter (T)? Did you see that? You may be thinking of only one intervention. If that is the case, you are comparing it with the baseline that already exists. However, you may want to compare two different interventions and measure the outcome between the two. So, logically, the O stands for outcome and the T stands for time. What outcome are you seeking to know more about? That is your O. In some literature, you will find there is no time element. More current writings typically include the T for good reason. You need an end point to your process in which you will measure your outcome and evaluate where to go next.

The next step that has already been alluded to is finding the evidence. Now, this part can become a bit overwhelming at times and sometimes frustrating. It may be overwhelming when you get thousands of results in your database search. It can be frustrating when you do not feel you are finding the right information or information within the past 5 years, which is typically the time definition of credible and scholarly work for evidence. The best advice here is to double-check your search terms. If you are getting way too much information, you need to narrow your search by using more defined terms. If you are not finding enough, there is usually one of two problems. You either have a very current and new topic that there is not much research available on or have the wrong search terms. That is all well and good, but you are probably wondering how to fix that when all the time you spent thinking led to those terms. You can keep trying, ask your faculty member for guidance, or seek the help of a librarian. Librarians are amazing and usually very helpful!

The third step in this process is to appraise the evidence. Again, this can feel daunting. You have all of these wonderful research articles and now you have to "appraise" them? What does that even mean? Well, it means that you have to determine whether it is from a trusted source, it has value, and it is relevant to your actual question. Occasionally, you start finding nuances in the research that create new questions and your thoughts and ideas can start to get a little muddy. You may start feeling a little lost. When you experience this, go back to your PICOT question and remind yourself of your focus.

One wonderful source of evidence for clinical questions in a database you may have access to through your university or even through some hospitals is UpToDate. This database provides a meta-analysis on various clinical problems. A meta-analysis is a type of systematic review that combines pertinent qualitative as well as quantitative data from multiple studies into one single conclusion. You could take the meta-analysis on your selected problem and search for the sources cited. Essentially, it does a considerable amount of work for you!

The next step is to apply the evidence. Now if you are researching a PICOT question in terms of writing a paper or doing a research project, you write up how the literature supports or justifies the intervention you have chosen. If you are applying this evidence to practice, you will integrate your findings into your clinical practice.

The fifth and final step in Strauss's (2005) process is to evaluate how you did with the previous steps. Were you effective? Were you efficient? How can you be more effective and efficient next time? I can honestly tell you, it takes practice to gain confidence in this process. However, the more you do it, the better you get and the easier it becomes.

Here is where some other models expand. For instance, Melnyk, Fineout-Overholt Stillwell, and Williamson (2010) continue the process by encouraging the need to disseminate the outcome of your work. It is very important to share the information and new knowledge we develop with others in our profession so that our body of evidence continues to grow and remain current. Sharing is also a hallmark of a profession that nursing has been working toward since the time of Florence Nightingale.

There are two other frequently cited evidence-based practice (EBP) models that break the process down into smaller steps while incorporating some change process steps. Like Melnyk, these two models also include dissemination as a final step. The first of these models is the Iowa Model Process by Titler et al. (2001). This model has 10 steps and includes a pilot of the change proposed to determine whether it should be fully adopted (Titler et al., 2001).

The second process is an EBP model developed at Johns Hopkins Nursing and is referred to as the PET Process. PET stands for the names of three phases. The first phase is the practice question and includes specific steps such as recruiting a team, developing the question, defining the scope of the question, assigning responsibility, and scheduling meetings (Dearholt & Dang, 2012). The second phase is the evidence stage that includes conducting a literature search, appraisal of the evidence, summarizing and synthesizing the evidence, and then developing the practice recommendation (Dearholt & Dang, 2012). With this process, you may not have a fully defined PICOT question to get you going, but rather let the literature define the intervention. Phase three of the PET process is translation. This stage includes determining fit, feasibility, and appropriateness of the intervention, creating an action plan, securing support, implementation, evaluation of outcomes, reporting to stakeholders, identifying future steps, and dissemination (Dearholt & Dang, 2012).

Remember, there are the five core steps to every process. The question becomes the following: Which process is best for you? Some provide a bit more change theory incorporated into the EBP process, whereas others remain true to the process itself. There is no right or wrong answer. The most important thing is that you are exploring, evaluating, implementing, and disseminating evidence.

CRITICAL THINKING QUESTIONS

1. Discuss one change you have initiated or fully implemented as a nurse. If you cannot think of one, search for a nurse-implemented change within a healthcare setting to discuss. How did you go about it? Did you have a process? Did it work? What would you do differently?

2. Think of a time when a change theory would help successfully implement a change. How would you do it?

3. Which change theory is most appealing to you? Do you think one is better than the others? How would you choose which one to use?

4. In thinking about different changes you have experienced in your work setting (either inside or outside of healthcare), do you think a change theory was used? Why or why not?

REFERENCES

American Association of Colleges of Nursing. (2011). The essentials of master's education in nursing. Retrieved from http://www.aacnnursing.org/Portals/42/Publications/MastersEssentials11.pdf

Best, M., & Neuhauser, D. (2006). Walter A Shewhart, 1924, and the Hawthorne factory. *Quality & Safety in Health Care, 15*(2), 142–143. doi:10.1136/qshc.2006.018093

Dearholt, S. L., & Dang, D. (2012). *Johns Hopkins nursing evidence-based practice: Model and guidelines* (2nd ed.). Indianapolis, IN: Sigma Theta Tau International.

Lally, P., van Jaarsveld, C. H. M., Potts, H. W. W., & Wardle, J. (2010). How are habits formed: Modelling habit formation in the real world. *European Journal of Social Psychology, 40*, 998–1009. doi:10.1002/ejsp.674

Lewin, K. (1947). Frontiers in group dynamics. In D. Cartwright (Ed.), *Field theory in social science*. London, UK: Social Science Paperbacks.

Longo, A. (2013). Change, complexity, and creativity. In L. Roussel (Ed.), *Management and leadership for nurse administrators* (pp. 121–161). Burlington, MA: Jones & Bartlett Learning.

Melnyk, B. M. (2005), Advancing evidence-based practice in clinical and academic settings. *Worldviews on Evidence-Based Nursing, 2*(3): 161–165. doi:10.1111/j.1741-6787.2005.00027.x

Melnyk, B. M., Fineout-Overholt, E., Stillwell, S. B., & Williamson, K. M. (2010). Evidence-based practice: Step by step: The seven steps of evidence-based practice. *American Journal of Nursing, 110*(1), 51–53. doi:10.1097/01.NAJ.0000366056.06605.d2

Moen, R. D., & Norman, C. L. (2010). Circling back: Clearing up myths about the Deming cycle and seeing how it keeps evolving. *Quality Progress,* 22–28. Retrieved from https://s3.amazonaws.com/wedi/www/FileManager/circling-back.pdf

Strauss, S. E. (2005). *Evidence-based medicine: How to practice and teach EBM* (3rd ed.). New York, NY: Churchill Livingstone.

Titler, M. G., Kleiber, C., Steelman, V., Rakel, B., Budreau, G., Everett, L. Q., … & Goode, C. J. (2001). The Iowa Model of evidence-based practice to promote quality care. *Critical Care Nursing Clinics of North America, 13*(4), 497–509.

12

AACN Essentials

Mindy Thompson and Annie Donaway

OBJECTIVES

1. Examine the competencies expected of the MSN-prepared nurse according to the MSN American Association of Colleges of Nursing (AACN) Essentials.

2. Review the competencies expected of the BSN-prepared nurse according to the BSN AACN Essentials.

3. Compare and contrast BSN- and MSN-prepared nurse competencies as defined by the AACN Essentials documents.

4. Describe differences between BSN and MSN competencies as defined by the AACN Essentials documents.

Something motivated you to return to school to seek a higher degree. Perhaps it was a particular job or position you wanted that requires at least a master's degree. Maybe it is a personal pursuit to achieve an MSN or even a terminal degree. Whatever it was that got you here, you may be wondering what the big difference is other than the obvious information you learn in your nursing classes that focused on a higher level of understanding in areas such as pharmacology, pathophysiology, and so forth. Any time you earn a higher degree, the level of contribution to the profession is expected to increase as well. In this chapter, we compare the AACN Essentials that delineate what is expected of a master's-prepared nurse as it compares with that of a baccalaureate-prepared nurse (BSN). Table 12.1 lists the competency categories identified by the AACN for

TABLE 12.1 Differences Between BSN and MSN Competencies

ESSENTIAL	BSN	MSN
I	Liberal education for baccalaureate generalist nursing practice	Background for practice from sciences and humanities
II	Basic organizational and systems leadership for quality care and patient safety	Organizational and systems leadership
III	Scholarship for evidence-based practice	Quality improvement and safety
IV	Information management and application of patient care technology	Translating and integrating scholarship into practice
V	Healthcare policy, finance, and regulatory environment	Informatics and healthcare technologies
VI	Interprofessional communication and collaboration for improving patient health outcomes	Health policy and advocacy for patients and populations
VII	Clinical prevention and population health	Interprofessional collaboration for improving patient and population health outcomes
VIII	Professionalism and professional values	Clinical prevention and population health for improving health
IX	Baccalaureate generalist nursing practice	Master's-level nursing practice

each degree. You will see how they are strikingly similar and each has one conceptual area different than the other. The baccalaureate essentials include competencies on professionalism because this is the ideal level of education one would enter into the profession (Institute of Medicine, 2000). Professionalism is not expanded on at the MSN level and quality improvement (QI) is added.

EDUCATIONAL BASIS

AACN BSN Essential I: Liberal Education for Baccalaureate Generalist Nursing Practice

AACN (2008) declares that a liberal education that includes study of the humanities, natural sciences, and social sciences allows for an appreciation of diversity. This appreciation then translates to both a greater ability to provide culturally sensitive and competent nursing care and the ability to be a collaborative member of the healthcare team. Skills gained through liberal arts education should include competencies in "inquiry, analysis, critical thinking, and communication" as well as "information technology, teamwork, and interprofessional problem solving" (AACN, 2008, p. 11). Cumulatively, a liberal arts foundation provides a solid base on which to build graduate-level education.

AACN MSN Essential I: Background for Practice From Sciences and Humanities

AACN (2011) distinguishes the academic difference between BSN and master's-prepared nurses (MSN) by the application of information. Whereas BSN-prepared nurses are key contributors and collaborators to the healthcare team, MSN-prepared nurses are expected to "fully analyze, design, implement, and evaluate nursing care" across a variety of patient populations in both clinical and community-based settings (AACN, 2011, p. 9). In addition to humanities, social sciences, and natural sciences, MSN-prepared nurses incorporate information from "biopsychosocial fields, genetics, public health, quality improvement (QI), health economics, translational science, and organizational sciences" to achieve continuous improvements (AACN, 2011, p. 9).

ORGANIZATIONAL AND SYSTEMS LEADERSHIP

AACN BSN Essential II: Basic Organizational and Systems Leadership for Quality Care and Patient Safety

AACN (2008) identifies the BSN role in systems leadership for quality care and patient safety to be primarily focused on the understanding of these concepts. BSN-prepared nurses should be able to assist with basic quality and safety processes and apply evidence-based information to their personal practice. In addition, they should be able to evaluate patient care within nursing science frameworks, taking contemporary culture, economic, organization, and political factors in consideration (AACN, 2008).

AACN MSN Essential II: Organizational and Systems Leadership

At the MSN-prepared level of nursing practice, the expectation is for nurses to promote quality and safety through key leadership skills (AACN, 2011). MSN-prepared nurses are equipped to build and leverage working relationships across interprofessional teams to coordinate patient care, implement conflict resolution strategies, and apply current evidence across patient care settings and continuums while assuming accountability for quality outcomes. They act as change agents at the system level while analyzing the impact of those systems on clients served.

EVIDENCE-BASED PRACTICE

AACN BSN Essential III: Scholarship for Evidence-Based Practice

AACN (2008) focuses Essential III on scholarship and evidence-based practice. At the BSN level, there are three main foci. These are identification of practice issues, evaluation and application of current evidence, and evaluation of outcomes (AACN, 2008). BSN-prepared nurses should have a basic understanding of the research process and be able to advocate for the protection of human subjects. With the ability to evaluate information for credibility, the BSN-prepared nurse collaborates with the healthcare team to apply evidence in combination with clinical judgment, interprofessional perspectives, and patient preferences to achieve improved patient outcomes (AACN, 2008). BSN-prepared nurses understand how healthcare quality and safety measures come to be through the research process and are equipped to propose solutions to practice issues that may negatively impact patient outcomes (AACN, 2008).

AACN MSN Essential IV: Translating and Integrating Scholarship into Practice

AACN (2011) makes a clear distinction between BSN and MSN in the area of scholarship. Whereas BSN-prepared nurses are well equipped to evaluate sources and apply evidence, MSN-prepared nurses are expected to integrate not only evidence but also theory, clinical judgment, and interprofessional perspectives to improve practice and patient groups or aggregates. Of course, MSN-prepared nurses should also support ethical processes for research including protection of human subjects. Working as a change agent, the MSN-prepared nurse should clearly communicate current evidence with credible sources across various audiences to inform practice as well as evaluate outcomes (AACN, 2011). BSN-prepared nurses should evaluate sources for credibility, whereas MSN-prepared nurses should critically appraise evidence to inform their own practice to disseminate into the profession, thereby having a much broader impact (AACN, 2011).

QUALITY

The topic of quality is incorporated into Essential II for the BSN. Quality is one area where MSN-prepared nurses are expected to directly contribute to an overall culture of safety while following high-reliability organization principles (Agency for Healthcare Research and Quality [AHRQ], 2017). The BSN role focuses more on a quality assurance process to ensure standards are met, whereas the MSN role is focused on the evaluation and development of continuous QI processes. Simply put, the BSN level of practice focuses on application and evaluation of quality and the MSN level of practice uses more advanced skills to disseminate evidence and synthesize information to improve organizational processes.

AACN MSN Essential III: Quality Improvement and Safety

The focus of the MSN-prepared nurse in Essential III is further on quality and the QI process. When evidence is combined with QI processes, trends can be analyzed and impacts on quality and safety can be quantified (AACN, 2011). MSN-prepared nurses not only integrate evidence into their own practice as a BSN-prepared nurse does but also analyze information and QI models to design systems and solutions (AACN, 2011). They engage in peer review, advocacy, error reporting, and professional contribution activities. This further aids in their ability to contribute to the six domains of healthcare quality (safe, effective, patient-centered, timely, efficient, and equitable) identified by the AHRQ as they lead QI initiatives that incorporate sociocultural factors that influence healthcare delivery (AACN, 2011; AHRQ, 2016).

INFORMATION, INFORMATICS, AND HEALTHCARE TECHNOLOGY

AACN BSN Essential IV: Information Management and Application of Patient Care Technology

Perhaps more important than the skills a BSN-prepared nurse has in the area of information management and technology is an attitude that en-courages, supports, and advocates for continual innovation and learning in the area of technology. BSN-prepared nurses should be able to use computer information systems (CIS) to communicate and collaborate with the healthcare team as well as document patient care with standardized terminology. They also use CIS to inform safe patient care delivery through data evaluation while maintaining "data security, regulatory requirements, confidentiality, and clients' right to privacy" (AACN, 2008, p. 20). BSN-prepared nurses also know that to successfully implement patient care technology, workflow and care processes should be evaluated for design first (AACN, 2008). They should also participate in the evaluation of CIS through policy and procedure revision and development processes within organizations (AACN, 2008).

AACN MSN Essential V: Informatics and Healthcare Technologies

According to the AACN (2011), informatics and healthcare technology encompasses five overarching themes. These are as follows:

1. Use of patient care and other technologies to deliver and enhance care

2. Communication technologies to integrate and coordinate care

3. Data management to analyze and improve outcomes of care

4. Health information management for evidence-based care and health education

5. Facilitation and use of electronic health records to improve patient care (p. 17)

MSN-prepared nurses should analyze technologies and evaluate data to assure patient safety, develop cost-effective strategies, and improve health outcomes (AACN, 2011). Just as all nurses are expected to maintain ethical practice, MSN-prepared nurses promote policies that embody those principles and standards. Whereas BSN-prepared nurses use patient care technology to document care, MSN-prepared nurses oversee and guide the integration of these technologies. They also use patient care technology and learning theories to instruct patients and others (AACN, 2011).

POLICY, FINANCE, REGULATION, AND ADVOCACY

AACN BSN Essential V: Healthcare Policy, Finance, and Regulatory Environment

BSN-prepared nurses are equipped with "basic knowledge of healthcare policy, finance, and regulatory environments, including local, state, national, and global healthcare trends" (AACN, 2008, p. 21). This knowledge enables understanding of the relationship between healthcare structure and financial implications through costs and reimbursements (AACN, 2008). From a policy standpoint, BSN-prepared nurses are able to investigate legislative and regulatory processes as they relate to healthcare while understanding state and national laws that define their practice (AACN, 2008). BSN nurses are able to correlate policy and procedure on organization, state, and federal levels to healthcare delivery and practice while advocating for those they serve (AACN, 2008). Being involved in political processes that would influence healthcare policy is an expectation of BSN-prepared nurses as stated by the AACN (2008).

AACN MSN Essential VI: Health Policy and Advocacy for Patients and Populations

When looking at the AACN list of competencies for MSN-prepared nurses in this area, the list is much shorter than that of the BSN. That is because the basic and core functions of nurses in the health policy arena are expected at the BSN level. However, at the MSN level, a deeper analysis of how policies impact healthcare, practice, and outcomes should occur (AACN, 2011). BSN nurses are expected to be involved in the political process of policy formation, whereas MSN nurses should contribute to policy development and implementation at organization, state, and federal levels (AACN, 2011). One highly impactful difference MSN nurses can make is to advocate for the public as well as the profession by disseminating evidence through the nursing perspective to policy makers as well as stakeholders (AACN, 2011). Both BSN- and MSN-prepared nurses have important roles in the policy-making and advocacy realms.

INTERPROFESSIONALISM AND OUTCOMES

AACN BSN Essential VI: Interprofessional Communication and Collaboration for Improving Patient Health Outcomes

AACN (2008) identifies the need for BSN-prepared nurses to recognize differences in scope, education, and licensure among other healthcare team members. This recognition allows for an increased understanding and ability to relate to those people whom nurses need to collaborate with to provide evidence-based, patient-centered care. Of course, any time there is a need to work with others, there will be opportunities to negotiate, manage and resolve conflict, and build positive relationships that BSN-prepared nurses should possess the skills to accomplish (AACN, 2008). Through working with others, BSN nurses should work to bring the nursing perspective to situations to support the goal of optimizing patient outcomes while functioning as a patient advocate (AACN, 2008).

AACN MSN Essential VII: Interprofessional Collaboration for Improving Patient and Population Health Outcomes

The competencies for MSN-prepared nurses in the area of population health are strikingly similar to those of the BSN at first glance (AACN, 2011). However, this is one area where the differences between the BSN and MSN roles actually have a much broader scope. The BSN-prepared nurses are expected to collaborate and work on patient outcomes within their immediate daily function. MSN-prepared nurses are expected to "intervene at the system level" to advocate for the nursing profession while also making positive impacts on patient care (AACN, 2011, p. 5). This intervention is done by acting as a leader in interprofessional environments and building partnerships while mentoring and coaching other nurses around them using knowledge and skills of team dynamics and group processes (AACN, 2011).

CLINICAL PREVENTION, HEALTH PROMOTION, AND POPULATION HEALTH

AACN BSN Essential VII: Clinical Prevention and Population Health

To work toward illness prevention and health promotion, nurses need to be able to evaluate both protective and predictive factors that include genetics at the individual, family, group, community, and population level (AACN, 2008). BSN nurses should be able to complete a thorough health history that includes genetic risks, beliefs, values, and attitudes (AACN, 2008). Once this information is obtained, BSN nurses use behavioral change techniques to instruct and guide clients to wellness. Of course, competencies from previous essentials such as collaboration, information technology, and so forth should also be used in this process (AACN, 2008).

BSNs participate and have skills in emergency preparedness that empower them to be very valuable in times of disaster, mass casualty, or other emergencies where entire populations are affected (AACN, 2008). BSNs are prepared to consider and evaluate available resources, resource allocation, "effectiveness, efficiency, cost-effectiveness, and equity" while advocating for social justice, vulnerable populations, and elimination of health disparities (AACN, 2008, p. 25).

AACN MSN Essential VIII: Clinical Prevention and Population Health for Improving Health

The MSN-prepared nurse builds on the BSN skills by incorporating multiple variants such as determinants of health, genetics, genomics, and epidemiologic data to administer and oversee evidence-based interventions to prevent illness and promote health (AACN, 2011). In addition, MSNs are well equipped to evaluate culturally responsive processes they design and implement using information technology and credible data sources (AACN, 2011). MSNs also incorporate information technology, nursing science, and scientific process skills to promote health policy, health education, communication strategies, and interventions (AACN, 2011).

PROFESSIONALISM AND PROFESSIONAL VALUE

AACN BSN Essential VIII: Professionalism and Professional Value

"Professionalism and the inherent values of altruism, autonomy, human dignity, integrity, and social justice are fundamental to the discipline of nursing" (AACN, 2008, p. 26). All nurses should embody and act out these values both in and out of their work environment. This is one essential that is listed in the BSN Essentials but not in the MSN Essentials simply because these are actions expected of all nurses and should occur at all nursing practice levels. With nurses being the most trusted professionals since 2001, nurses are known for moral, ethical, and legal conduct in both personal and professional behavior (AACN, 2008; Brenan, 2017). Nurses promote the image of nursing by demonstrating professionalism in their appearance, actions, and attention to professional boundaries (AACN, 2008). They spend time reflecting on evaluating their own beliefs and how those beliefs affect the care they are able to provide to others. When there is a conflict with a nurse's ability to provide unbiased care to a patient, family, group, or population, they must communicate that bias to then become an advocate (AACN, 2008).

Advocacy happens on multiple levels in various ways. Nurses advocate for clients by protecting confidentiality, working to resolve ethical dilemmas, and inhibiting unsafe, illegal, or unethical practices (AACN, 2008). Of course, all nurses are interested and pursue the continual growth of their own knowledge, skill, and development on personal and professional levels. They recognize the connection between their own health and well-being and their ability to provide sustainable quality care to those they serve (AACN, 2008).

NURSING PRACTICE

AACN BSN Essential IX: Baccalaureate Generalist Nursing Practice

BSN nurses provide comprehensive and focused assessments that are developmentally and culturally appropriate. They acknowledge a connection between genetics and genomics to health and outcomes as patient-centered, holistic care is implemented. They understand "human growth and development, pathophysiology, pharmacology, medical management, and nursing management across the health–illness continuum, across the life span, and in all healthcare settings" (AACN, 2008, p. 31). They communicate effectively with patients, families, and the healthcare team to implement care that respects patient and family wishes and manage conflict when it arises throughout the life span (AACN, 2008). BSN-prepared nurses teach patients and families with appropriate methods to satisfy developmental stage, age, culture, spirituality, learner preferential style, and health literacy considerations (AACN, 2008). Evidence-based and patient-centered practice is used to treat both acute and chronic patients in all settings and through multiple functional problems, including frequently occurring geriatric syndromes (AACN, 2008). BSN-prepared nurses support care transitions that include discharge planning (AACN, 2008).

Nurses provide an environment where safe care can be provided to obtain high-quality patient outcomes and revise plans of care as needed on the basis of ongoing evaluations (AACN, 2008). BSNs possess both psychomotor and clinical reasoning skills to manage patient care while also supervising other healthcare team members (AACN, 2008). They have an introductory understanding of complementary and alternative treatments (AACN, 2008). BSNs realize how healthcare professionals' spiritual beliefs and values impact care they provide (AACN, 2008). BSN-prepared nurses understand their role in emergency preparedness as well as environmental factors that pose a risk (AACN, 2008). Two additional BSN competencies are the ability to develop therapeutic nurse–patient relationships and the ability to tolerate ambiguity and unpredictability not only in the world but also within healthcare systems and teams (AACN, 2008).

AACN MSN Essential IX: Master's-Level Nursing Practice

Scientific and ethical principles provide the basis to all nursing practice. Whereas BSN-prepared nurses conduct comprehensive and focused assessments, MSN-prepared nurses complete comprehensive and systematic assessments to apply current and credible evidence to practice nursing (AACN, 2011). They also act as "advocate[s] for patients, families, caregivers, communities, and members of the healthcare team" as they use information and communication technology to support outcomes (AACN, 2011, p. 27). They enact leadership skills to teach, coach, and mentor others (AACN, 2011). MSN nurses analyze data related to epidemiology, social factors, and environment as well as skills in economics, business, and systems to design, implement, and evaluate nursing activities (AACN, 2011). Nurses at this level use learning and teaching theories to design, deliver, and evaluate education provided to individuals or groups in a variety of settings (AACN, 2011). They work to build therapeutic relationships that allows leverage to negotiate "patient-centered, culturally appropriate, evidence-based goals and modalities of care" (AACN, 2011, p. 28). Although all nurses should be lifelong learners, MSNs should have an evolving personal philosophy of nursing during their pursuit of continual growth and development (AACN, 2011). BSNs are participants and contributors to the interdisciplinary healthcare team, whereas MSNs participate, contribute, and lead those teams to improve and promote optimal outcomes for patients, families, groups, and populations.

CRITICAL THINKING QUESTIONS

1. Which MSN Essential are you most surprised by?

2. After reading this chapter, is the difference between BSN- and MSN-level nursing consistent with what you imagined? Why or why not?

3. Are there any of the MSN Essentials that you are apprehensive about? Which one(s) and why?

4. Are there any of the BSN Essentials you feel you could work on being more effective before progressing to the MSN Essential? Which one(s) and why?

REFERENCES

Agency for Healthcare Research and Quality. (2016). The six domains of health care quality. Retrieved from https://www.ahrq.gov/professionals/quality-patient-safety/talkingquality/create/sixdomains.html

Agency for Healthcare Research and Quality. (2017). Patient safety primer: High reliability. Retrieved from https://psnet.ahrq.gov/primers/primer/31/high-reliability

American Association of Colleges of Nursing. (2008). The essentials of baccalaureate education for professional nursing practice. Retrieved from http://www.aacnnursing.org/Portals/42/Publications/BaccEssentials08.pdf

American Association of Colleges of Nursing. (2011). The essentials of master's education in nursing. Retrieved from http://www.aacnnursing.org/Portals/42/Publications/MastersEssentials11.pdf

Brenan, M. (2017). Nurses keep healthy lead as most honest, ethical profession. *Gallup News*. Retrieved from http://news.gallup.com/poll/224639/nurses-keep-healthy-lead-honest-ethical-profession.aspx?g_source=CATEGORY_SOCIAL_POLICY_ISSUES&g_medium=topic&g_campaign=tiles

Institute of Medicine. (2000). *To err is human: Building a safer health system.* Washington, DC: National Academies Press.

13

Interprofessional Collaboration

Brenda Scott

OBJECTIVES

1. Identify the roles of the MSN-prepared nurse in interprofessional collaboration.
2. Determine strategies to engage others in interprofessional collaboration.
3. Examine challenges that may arise when participating in interprofessional collaboration.
4. Evaluate the need for shared goals when participating in interprofessional collaboration.
5. Develop strategies to navigate candid conversations.

Have you ever had a moment where you dreamed of being stranded on a deserted island with no help, while trying to care for the most critical patient? No? Well neither have most of us. As nurses, we seek to work in places where we feel comfortable, safe, supported, and part of a team. We know that the shift goes better when we have coworkers around us to provide support and guidance. Many situations occur in the various healthcare settings that require the work of an interprofessional team. Think of care coordination meetings, disaster drills, receiving lab results, and the list goes on with respect to times a team is needed to support an outcome.

The American Nurses Association (2015) defines interprofessional collaboration (IC) as "integrated enactment of knowledge, skills, and values and attitudes that define working together across the professions, with other health care workers, and with patients, along with families and communities, as appropriate to improve health outcomes." As a nurse, it is important to identify the key players who can best assist you in a given circumstance. If you are working at the bedside to provide care to a laboring mother, your interprofessional team will be different from that of the disaster professional working to prepare a facility for response to a tornado.

The American Association of Colleges of Nursing (AACN) Essentials of Master's Education in Nursing includes IC as one of the expectations within all MSN educational programs. You can review the AACN Essentials within Chapter 12.

Collaboration is key to ensure that outcomes are met. The Institute of Medicine (IOM, 2011) recommends that "nurses should be full partners, with physicians and other healthcare professionals, in redesigning health care in the United States" (p. 29). The IOM identifies several strategies to accomplish this including putting patients first, commitments from organizational leadership that IC is seen as a priority, and that all practitioners' contributions are valued, and effective team communication is valued and modeled (2011).

INTERPROFESSIONAL COLLABORATION STAKEHOLDERS

The Agency for Healthcare Research and Quality (AHRQ) has defined stakeholders "as persons or groups that have a vested interest in a clinical decision and the evidence that supports that decision." The stakeholders or key players will vary given the situation. If we are creating a new policy, the stakeholders may be nurses, doctors, patients, policy makers, and various other members of the healthcare team. If we are creating a facility disaster response plan, the stakeholders include facility emergency preparedness teams, city or county emergency managers, department leadership, fire departments, police departments, emergency medical services, community leaders, community members, public health professionals, and anyone else who would be involved in the response. Now, let's take this to the bedside. If you are the nurse working in a medical–surgical unit caring for a postoperative patient, who do you consider your stakeholders? You would consider your patient, their family, and the provider, but who else would you consider? Would you consider the lab technician and staffs of the departments of radiology, respiratory, physical therapy (PT), dietary, infection control, case management, and so on as stakeholders? These may all be key players or stakeholders in your patient's care and outcome. When you need lab results, you usually reach out to the laboratory and not the PT department. You reach out to the subject matter expert able to assist in your specific situation. The same type of process works when you consider stakeholders or key players in IC.

As a master's-prepared nurse, you will likely find yourself with a need to bring together and sometimes lead an interprofessional team. When you are working to create this team, you will identify stakeholders or key players. Who do you want at the table? You will need to work to identify the subject matter experts (SMEs). You will ensure that these experts are able to help you meet expected outcomes. Something else to consider when identifying stakeholders is separating management from leadership. As we all know, just because someone has a title does not make the person a leader. Often, a manager relies on his or her authority and power to make decisions and implement change, whereas a leader relies on influence and relationships. When considering stakeholders, especially to design and implement change, it is important to identify and engage both groups. It is also very important to never forget that the end user who will be impacted, including the patient, is a stakeholder as well.

TEAM DEVELOPMENT

Building a cohesive team dedicated to a purpose is difficult. Every member of the team has his or her own visible and hidden agendas and an idea of what success looks like (and that is not a bad thing as you accept this going into meetings). In 1965, psychologist and researcher, Bruce Tuckman identified group dynamics in four stages: forming–storming–norming–performing (Tuckman, 1965). In 1977, a fifth stage was identified: adjourning (Tuckman & Jensen, 1977). It is important to understand that these stages may occur in any order and may be reoccurring. Let's look at each of these stages.

Forming

The first step of team development is forming a team. This step is one of the most challenging and takes thoughtful deliberation. As we discussed in the section "Interprofessional Collaboration Stakeholders," making sure you have the needed team members to be successful is one of the biggest challenges. Even when you know the team members, there is still a forming period, although the more team members collaborate and trust, the shorter the period. During this time, members begin sharing backgrounds and interests and form impressions of each other. One of the most important pieces of the forming process is developing roles, goals, expectations, and so on. During this initial period, team members are highly dependent on the team leader to set the tone and guide them until assignments are given.

As a master's-prepared nurse, you may be called upon to lead teams. When identifying your goals and needs of a project, it is important to remember that others may have their own goals, ideas, or needs as well. This is where the visible and hidden agendas should be identified, explored, and weighed for value and merit. Just because someone has his or her own ideas or goals does not mean that collaboration cannot occur. During this phase, you might consider opportunities to get to know people better by using tools such as a motivational analysis tool. This tool can help you determine whether a person is motivated by achievement, influence and power, or affiliation with others (Mackenzie & Moore, 1993). This will help you identify how to talk to and gain success out of each team member. The next step is the storming phase.

Storming

The storming phase is one of the most complicated and necessary phases of team development. This phase requires patience, diligence, understanding, and a positive attitude. In this phase, members of the team will go through positive and negative experiences while they try to learn to work together. There will be issues in this phase as team members work to embrace roles, share ideas and expectations, and identify and challenge each other's opinions and working and learning styles until trust and collaboration are established. This stage can be a very uncertain time for teams that have not worked together before. Sadly, many teams fail in this stage and never progress or do not take the time to successfully come together and have a negative experience throughout the project. As the leader, you can help move the team forward to a more positive experience and outcome.

Norming

In the norming phase, everything begins to click together for the change agent as well as the team he or she is leading. This is the phase where the team members begin to work together as one, accept the roles they have been assigned, and work toward achieving the same goals. During this phase, team members begin to form both personal and professional relationships with each other and work toward goals that are mutually beneficial. You may also find yourself wanting to step back and let the team work toward solving problems, and that is okay. Once you have gone through all of the effort, frustration, time, and challenges of getting to norming, you might think you are done, all is well, and you can kick up your feet and relax. Not so fast.

Performing

Once the team has gelled and is working with a common purpose, the team has to perform. In the performing phase, teams work autonomously. As a leader of an interprofessional team, one of the most challenging activities sometimes is to release control given as a manager (or a leader on paper) and instead become a mentor investing time and energy in others. Throughout the previous phases, management and the ability to get things done was the glue that helped to bring things together. Now, skill in management shifts into leadership. During this phase, the delegation of work, new activity, and responsibility becomes the primary activity for a team leader. Just like in nursing, you can delegate tasks to unlicensed providers or team members, but you have to be confident in the team member's competency to perform the task at hand. The leader has already identified the competency level of team members in prior phases. Now, the leader must set expectations and provide coaching, mentoring, and professional development to team members as needed. This leadership will help team members maintain and exceed both personal and provided expectations. Shifting focus to team members allows for the sustainability of a well-rounded and high-functioning team, which is what should occur in this phase.

Adjourning

One of the hardest phases of team performance is adjourning. You know that feeling you get when you have taken care of a patient for a while and is now going home or a student who is about to graduate and your job in preparing him or her for entry into nursing is complete? That is what we are looking at during adjourning. In this phase, the team has finished its primary role and has met its objectives. Now, the decision is what to do with the team. Does the team move to another project? Does the team dissolve? All of these questions are challenging and may or may not be answered by the team leader. Sometimes, the institution may decide that a team needs to be reorganized. Adjourning is a challenging time for people who enjoy close relationships and are motivated by affiliation. One of the important aspects of this step is to ensure that the work and lessons learned are captured, and that the relationships are maintained.

KEY CONSIDERATIONS DURING INTERPROFESSIONAL COLLABORATION

Communication

Communication is the one thing that can make or break any process, project, or team. When considering interprofessional collaboration, communication will need to be a priority. As you are planning your project, you will want to consider who all needs to be part of it. Some common questions to ask yourself are as follows:

- Who will I need to provide regular updates?
- What information will I need to share?
- What information will the stakeholder need to be successful as a participant?
- What is the ideal method of communication?
- How transparent can I be with the entire project?
- What is the purpose? (Why?)

When you are forming an interprofessional team, you will need to consider the needs of each participant. For example, you will not communicate with someone from the health department the same way you will with the mayor of the town. These two participants have differing backgrounds and will need information presented to them in different ways. Communication styles are a huge consideration for all participants in the interprofessional team.

Conflict Resolution

Let's be honest, nobody gets along with everyone all the time. Sometimes we encounter conflict within our team. As an MSN-prepared nurse, you will commonly find yourself as the leader of IC. It will be important for you to develop skills to handle conflict resolution. The more you consider your response to conflict, the more you will be prepared for when the challenge arises. Three considerations for conflict resolution are reviewed as follows.

Candid Conversations

You may have heard candid conversations referred to as crucial conversations or high-stakes conversations. These conversations may occur at many points during IC. I think we would be remiss if we approached any interprofessional collaboration opportunity thinking we could avoid all types of conversation. The key is to be prepared. Although you may not be able to plan for every single detail or type of occurrence, it is a good idea to have a general idea about the process you will take to address the concerns.

After several years of practice, I have a process that I usually follow. The first step is to remove all of my personal feelings. In a high-stakes conversation, you cannot function on the basis of feelings. It is extremely difficult to remove your emotions when you are working on a project in which you are passionate. My personal practice is to leave my feelings at the door before approaching any type of IC. The truth is that the purpose of the IC has nothing to do with me as a person. You have to ask yourself: What is the goal of the conversation? What are we working toward as a group?

Mindfulness

One important aspect of IC interactions is to be aware that everyone brings a different perspective to the group. According to Ludwig & Kabat-Zinn (2008), "mindfulness involves attending to relevant aspects of experience in a nonjudgmental manner." It is important to be present in every situation. This is even more important in IC and candid conversations. The ability to remove all emotions, judgment, and assumptions from your response allows you to enter a conversation ready to hear the person you are engaging. When you can truly "hear" what another person is saying, it allows you to become a stronger leader. Recognizing that each individual brings their own perspective to the table and that each has value is a key leadership competency. Mindfulness in every interaction allows even the toughest conversations to feel a little less personal while adding value to each participant.

Resolution

When candid conversations occur, we are all working toward a resolution. The challenge presented is whether that resolution can be mutual for all involved. Mutual resolution is especially important in IC. One method to achieve resolution is the "CRIB" method (Patterson, Greeny, McMillan, and Switzler, 2002, pp. 83–87). These authors define the CRIB method as follows:

- C: Commit to seek mutual purpose.
- R: Recognize the purpose behind the strategy.
- I: Invent a mutual purpose.
- B: Brainstorm new strategies.

There is a recurrent theme found within this process of finding common ground.

The first step requires a commitment from all parties to stay engaged in the conversation no matter what. This is sometimes very difficult. Think about the following example: Let's say you are caring for a 99-year-old gentleman who has been diagnosed with end-stage renal disease. The patient has been on dialysis for many years. He has recently been admitted to the hospital following a fall and recent diagnosis of a hip fracture. He has been scheduled for surgery tomorrow. The patient verbalizes to you that he wishes to stop all treatment. His words: "I've lived a good life and I just need to rest now." His daughter is at his bedside. She verbalizes her wishes to do everything we can to "save Daddy." Can you see how this could present a situation where finding common ground would be difficult? What challenges will this nurse face? Can you see the ethical dilemma flags flying? I would challenge you to consider that there is an easy goal to work toward. We are all focused on what is best for the patient, right? The "common ground" for this scenario may be identifying what is best for the patient right now. This may be the mutual purpose identified as the first step in the CRIB method. The key is to stay in the discussion until you can reach this common ground. It would be easy for the patient to give in to the daughter's request because he does not want to anger her. It would be very easy for the daughter to overlook her father's request because she just wants more time with him. Commonly, we take the easy way out: Let's just make a decision and move on. When we are dealing with candid conversations in IC, it is important to be committed to the main goal. Although this patient scenario presents challenges, we can see the CRIB process in action. Reflect back on a time where you were involved in IC. Were there candid conversation that occurred? Was everyone involved in the candid conversation committed to finding that common ground? Have you been engaged in a candid conversation where you gave in just to move the project forward knowing it was not the right thing to do? Let's admit it is easier to avoid than to be committed to the conversation and process of finding common ground. Commit to staying in those hard, uncomfortable conversations and finding a common ground.

Let's continue with the same scenario. The second step in the CRIB process is to determine a strategy. Let's see how this applies to the scenario and then to IC.

We have seen the father, daughter, and nurse commit to the conversation until they find a common ground: Improve the situation. Do you see how this commitment is not agreeing with either side explicitly? We will get to a resolution eventually. Within the second step of CRIB, we need to gather more information. According to Patterson et al. (2002), one thing to consider is what each person wants versus the purpose (p. 87). We are going to see purpose popping up throughout this chapter. This is the "why" behind what we do. Why do they want what they want? What is the purpose?

It is easy for us, as nurses, to jump to conclusions when considering purpose. We have a lot of experience that we bring to the table, but that does not mean we always know the true "why" behind the situation. It can be easy to think the daughter is selfish and she just wants what she thinks is best for her. We may never consider that she was reunited with her father only 3 years ago after being adopted. Maybe she is requesting more time so she can build memories she never had. We can never assume we know the full story. So how does this apply to IC?

When working collaboratively, each stakeholder has a different set of knowledge, skills, and attitudes (KSAs) that he or she brings to the table. As leaders, we have to consider each toolbox, if you will, that each of these stakeholders brings with him or her. We also must consider the purpose bringing each participant to the team. Why are they involved? What is their level of commitment? Someone who has millions of dollars riding on the success of the IC and a personal purpose relating to the topic may have more passion than someone who was told to be there because his or her manager could not attend. In bedside nursing, we see something similar. Back to the scenario, you are caring for your patient and need lab results. Your purpose is to ensure that your patient receives quality care while improving the status of his health. You call the lab and are told your results will be available in an hour. You have a decision to make here. Do you request the lab technician to put yours first or do you take a step back and consider the purpose? You are focusing on your one patient. The lab technician is responsible for lab results for the entire facility. You probably find yourself asking: Is it the difference between life and death? If it is, you might choose to respond differently than if it is just a routine lab result. The important thing to remember here is to ask yourself about the purpose.

According to Patterson et al. (2002), the third component is to "invent a mutual purpose" (p. 87). Although in our scenario we have found differing purposes, this is commonly what you will see in IC. You commonly see your stakeholders involved for different reasons. Maybe you are involved because someone told you to be, maybe it is because you want to climb the clinical ladder, maybe it is because you have a personal goal that aligns, or maybe you just find yourself in the right place at the right time. No matter the reason, we all are motivated by different things. When we are dealing with candid conversations, we have to put our personal feelings aside and ask ourselves what the goal is.

In the patient scenario, the goal is to improve the current situation. Each stakeholder has a different route to achieve improvement. If they cannot agree on the small purpose (i.e., all treatments vs. no treatment), they can work to identify a broader purpose or goal. In this scenario, your broader goal is to work toward improving the current situation.

The final step is where the fun happens. The final step is to "brainstorm new strategies" (Patterson et al., 2002, p. 87) to allow for work toward a resolution. In the patient scenario, you may never get the daughter to agree to stop all treatment and you may never get the patient to accept all treatment, but an agreement can occur on certain aspects that satisfy each stakeholder. For example, the patient may agree to surgery correcting the fracture, whereas the daughter agrees to no longer receiving dialysis. Can you see this coming together?

How does this all apply to IC? Let's take a common nursing scenario and see how the CRIB method works. Think back to the scenario provided earlier about calling for lab results for your patient. Although you are concerned about your patient, the lab technician needs to consider the entire facility's priorities. As the nurse, you have to commit to staying in the discussion to reach a mutual purpose (C). Once you determine that both of you are on the same page or purpose, you can move to the next step. You have the conversation with the lab technician explaining why you will need the lab results quickly, as your patient's status is declining (R). Both of you have agreed that you want to serve patients and ensure that no patient suffers, so you have arrived at the "mutual purpose" (I). Now the fun begins, brainstorming ideas of how to meet at this mutual purpose. One solution might be for you to draw the blood and the lab technician will pick it up and provide results (B).

It is important to consider how this method can apply to those difficult relationships or opportunities where IC may be strained. Let's consider a budget conversation. You are the manager of a medical–surgical unit. You are entering a discussion with the chief financial officer and chief nursing officer to discuss your annual budget. As the manager, you are considering a point in the conversation where the CRIB method could be used. Pull out a blank piece of paper and reflect on how you will respond during each phase of the CRIB method. Be sure to consider strategies you may use in difficult times.

Reflection

Another important aspect of any IC is reflection. Have you ever had a moment where in your mind you resemble Superman, but when you look in the mirror this is not exactly what you see? The same can happen with self-reflection. It is important to pause and reflect on various situations. This is even more important in IC. Emotional intelligence (EI) has been a hot topic for years and self-reflection is one of the key components of people having high EI.

You likely are part of an interprofessional team because you bring subject matter expertise (SME) to the situation. You may not have been invited to participate if you did not have KSAs that apply to the goal to which the team is working toward. Even with your expertise, it is crucial to remain aware of your actual abilities. In other words, you cannot become arrogant. Have you seen arrogant people? They always know the best way to do things, have the best response, and usually have little room for input from others. This is why self-reflection is imperative in personal and professional settings. If you develop consistent self-reflection practices, you can avoid becoming one of those arrogant people.

There are many self-reflection practices that you can incorporate in your daily practice. One common practice is writing a reflection. You may have experience with journaling. When self-reflecting using journaling, I like to ask myself three main questions:

1.   Did I meet my goal(s)?

2.   If I could go back and do it again, what would I change?

3.   What resources or new learnings could have made me better in this experience?

Another option for reflection is to dialogue with others. Dialoguing is where you find and engage the person that you trust most and talk through things. This person should be someone who speaks honestly with you—does not just tell you what you want to hear—and may be the person you consider your mentor. The same three questions, as stated earlier, can be used in this reflection opportunity. The key here is to walk away with information to use when conducting an internal reflection of the situation.

Mindfulness was addressed earlier in the chapter. It is a key piece in self-reflection. These two concepts truly go hand in hand. In nursing, we are typically in situations impacting more than ourselves. We are caring for patients and their families, and interacting with colleagues. As we interact with people who may not see things exactly as we do, we must be mindful of their perspective. Mindfulness becomes an important aspect of reflection.

Another type of reflection includes group reflection. One method of achieving group reflection is through participation in "hot washes." Although the origin of the term traces to the military and has a minimally documented history, hot washes are meetings that occur immediately following an exercise, event, or activity. These meetings can serve as either a formal or an informal type of reflection, depending on design, to review what went well, what needs improvement, and what needs immediate correction. How well attended a hot wash is and how diverse the population is can impact the success. The hot wash offers an informal opportunity to reflect as a group on the following:

1.   Successes that should be captured and continued as best practice

2.   Things that maybe went okay or not so well and need to be tweaked to move them toward best practice and success

3.   A forum to address action that requires immediate correction and change

If there was a recent issue regarding patient and employee safety, it would be wise to have the safety and security leads in the hot wash.

The hot wash process may also lead the host and participants to think about future planning efforts and changes. Another thing groups typically discover is that the right people are often not in the room during the hot wash. By using the hot wash as an opportunity for IC, nurses can improve their relationships, planning, and capabilities working with other internal and external stakeholders. By having multiple inputs from a variety of stakeholders, you may see things that may have been missed otherwise. This is an opportunity for collaboration and problem solving.

You may also be familiar with debriefing as a means of reflection. Debriefing is very similar to the hot wash process. You may be most familiar with debriefing after a clinical or simulation experience (National League of Nursing, 2015). Debriefing allows you to discuss practice and process with an SME. Reflect on your postclinical debrief session with your clinical instructor. Commonly in debriefing, we are asking each student to reflect on what went well and what did not work so well.

In group reflection, both hot washes and debriefing, immediate corrections are identified to address safety issues. In hot washes, there is usually a time period immediately following where a full improvement plan is created addressing all issues identified. In debriefing, you may cover all necessary changes and may even repeat the experience.

ROLE OF THE MSN-PREPARED NURSE

We have discussed things to consider during IC, so next we identify the role of the MSN-prepared nurse. Generally speaking, as your level of education increases, so does your responsibility. Even in times without a managerial title, coworkers may look to you for guidance and best practices. So, what is your role in IC? There are a few to consider: SME, change agent, and leader.

Subject Matter Expertise

With the advanced degree comes more subject matter expertise. Think back to your first nursing degree and reflect at how much you have grown professionally since that time. Although you probably are not an expert in all areas, you do hold a certain level of expertise on many topics. When you are part of the IC team, you will bring KSAs to the opportunity. It is important to always stay in touch with your abilities. Consider the opportunity to participate in IC as a means to acknowledge the KSAs you demonstrate. You must also consider what others are bringing to the team.

As we have seen throughout this chapter, it is important to have the right people at the table at the right time. When you are creating a disaster plan for your organization, you would not want only your chief nursing officer and the chief financial officer at the table. You would want all stakeholders involved with the subject matter expertise to ensure that your facility is truly prepared to respond. The same goes for a code blue situation. You do not want only the admissions clerk in the room. No, you want healthcare professionals trained cardiopulmonary resuscitation (CPR) in advanced cardiac life support (ACLS). Do you see how SMEs can improve the outcomes of a situation? This is the same for the MSN-prepared nurse. Identify your KSAs and what you can bring to the table, and then, position yourself to engage in IC on the basis of those KSAs. This positioning will allow you to function as an SME and ultimately improve outcomes.

Change Agent

The MSN-prepared nurse can be involved in major changes. The nurse must identify the KSAs or SMEs that are brought to the IC team. The charge of the MSN-prepared nurse is to become the change agent. The focus of the change agent is to improve outcomes. See Chapter 11 for more on change agents.

Leader

Many times, MSN-prepared nurses will find themselves in a position of leadership. Although this role does not always come with a title, the responsibility is there. Remember that a leader is someone people want to follow. This role is very different than that of a manager people must follow because of the title. Even without a title, you have an opportunity to create an environment and practice in which others want to follow. Leaders work to influence change, title or not.

Do you see how becoming aware of your SME and KSAs can help you become a leader to influence change? Can you think of a scenario that requires IC in which you can function as a leader for change while acting as the SME?

CASE STUDY

You are leading a team in the emergency department (ED) in a project focused on improving patient outcomes. This project requires the participation of nursing, pharmacy, laboratory, and the ED director. In this project, nursing is focused on improving the outcomes of the patient while managing the workload of the nurses. The pharmacy team representative is focused on this as well, but sees an opportunity to implement stronger protocols that will result in a larger amount of certain medications being kept in the automated medication dispensing system and accessible to nursing and medical staff. The laboratory team representative sees an opportunity to combine labs and reduce the number of lab orders requiring processing by his or her team. The ED director sees this as an opportunity to decrease staffing needs and increase reimbursement opportunities. Answer the following questions:

1. Who are the stakeholders in this project?
2. How can you use the "CRIB" method?
3. What KSAs do you bring to the table?
4. How can you act as the change agent?
5. What are ways you can lead this project without having a title?
6. How will you use personal reflection?
7. How will group reflection benefit this project?

REFERENCES

American Nurses Association. (2015). *Nursing: Scope and standards of practice* (3rd ed.). Silver Spring, MD: Author.

Institute of Medicine. (2011). *The future of nursing: Leading change, advancing health.* Washington, DC: National Academies Press.

Ludwig, D. S., & Kabat-Zinn, J. (2008). Mindfulness in medicine. *JAMA: Journal of the American Medical Association, 100*(11), 1350–1352. doi:10.1001/jama.300.11.1350

Mackenzie, M., & Moore, G. (1993). *The volunteer development toolbox: Tools and techniques to enhance volunteer and staff effectiveness.* Darien, IL: Heritage Arts Publishing.

National League of Nursing. (2015). Interprofessional collaboration in education and practice: A living document from the National League for Nursing. *NLN VisionSeries.* Retrieved from http://www.nln.org/docs/default-source/default-document-library/ipe-ipp-vision.pdf?sfvrsn=14

Nunez, L. (2015). Achieving quality and improved outcomes through interprofessional collaboration. Retrieved from https://www.asha.org/Articles/Achieving-Quality-and-Improved-Outcomes-Through-Interprofessional-Collaboration/

Patterson, K., Greeny, J., McMillan, R., & Switzler, A. (2002). *Crucial conversations: Tools for talking when stakes are high* (2nd ed.). New York, NY: McGraw-Hill Education.

Sullivan, M., Kiovsky, R. D., Mason, D. J., Hill, C. D., & Dukes, C. (2015). Interprofessional collaboration and education: Working together to ensure excellence in healthcare. *American Journal of Nursing, 115*(3), 47–54. doi:10.1097/01. NAJ.0000461822.40440.58

Tuckman, B. W. (1965). Development sequence in small groups. *Psychological Bulletin*, *63*(6), 384–399. doi:10.1037/h0022100

Verhaegh, K. J., Seller-Boersma, A., Simons, R., Steenbruggen, J., Geerlings, S. E., de Rooij, S. E., & Buurman, B. M. (2017). An exploratory study of healthcare professionals' perceptions of interprofessional communication and collaboration. *Journal of Care*, *31*(3), 397–400. doi:10.1080/13561820.2017.1289158

SECTION V

Special Topics

In this section, we take a look at some special topics in nursing. All nurses are responsible for lifelong learning. In Chapter 14, we discuss doctoral education and options related to terminal nursing degrees. Of course, there are other terminal degree options such as doctorates in education, management, informatics, and many more. The focus in Chapter 14 is on those options with a nursing focus. In Chapter 15, we take a look at caring for yourself as you care for others. The health of healthcare workers has been an area for improvement for a number of years, so we dig into this topic and offer insight and suggestion. Finally, in Chapter 16, we discuss mentoring in terms of giving and receiving as well as outcomes of positive mentoring experiences.

14

Special Topics: Considerations for Lifelong Learning

Gina M. Oliver

OBJECTIVES

1. Identify options to continue education.
2. Define lifelong learning.
3. Differentiate the types of certification.
4. Discuss how nurses may obtain continuing education units (CEUs).
5. Explain what activities may be considered self-directed learning.

As you have noticed from being a registered nurse, learning never stops. Obtaining a master's degree does not end the need for lifelong learning. You will continue to need to explore healthcare research and keep abreast of the new knowledge in our profession. Lifelong learning can be accomplished through several avenues, including formal and informal paths. There is always more to learn, and as nurses, we should always be eager to learn more.

DEFINITION

Lifelong learning may be defined as "the activities people perform throughout their life to improve their knowledge, skills, and competence in a particular field" (Koper & Tattersall, 2004, p. 689). Lifelong learning entails the learner setting goals and choosing methods to acquire the knowledge and skills required to meet those goals (Collins, 2009). Davis, Taylor, and Reyes (2014) found that the qualities of a lifelong learner in nursing are "reflection, questioning, enjoying learning, understanding the dynamic nature of knowledge, and engaging in learning by actively seeking learning opportunities" (p. 444). This type of learning is significantly different than when you went to elementary or secondary school and everything you learned was predetermined by your teachers.

TERMINAL DEGREE OPTIONS

Earning a master's degree in nursing is a laudable effort and should be commended for increasing your knowledge level; however, you may want to consider expanding your formal education with earning a terminal degree. The terminal degree in nursing is a doctoral degree. In the past, nurses obtained a doctorate in other disciplines such as education, psychology, or anthropology, to name a few. There are still some nurses today who prefer to obtain their doctorate in a discipline outside of nursing, but now that there are many nursing programs that offer doctoral programs, the majority of nurses are obtaining their terminal degrees in nursing.

There are two main nursing doctorates, the doctor of philosophy (PhD) and the doctor of nursing practice (DNP). The PhD is a research-focused degree in which nurse scientists create new knowledge in nursing also known as applied research. The curriculum focuses primarily on theory, research design and methodology, and statistics (Hicks & Patterson, 2017). Students complete a dissertation, which is a research project designed, implemented, and evaluated by the student with the assistance of a faculty mentor.

The DNP is a practice-focused degree in the advanced practice or leadership roles. The curriculum focuses on the selected advanced nursing role as well as translation of nursing research. This means taking applied research and implementing it in a selected area applicable to the advanced doctoral role. Students complete a scholarly project to improve health outcomes or make improvements in a health system.

CHOOSING A DOCTORAL PROGRAM

Choosing the correct doctoral program for you can be a complex process. The first step is to decide whether you wish to create new knowledge for the nursing profession and obtain a research doctorate (PhD) or pursue a clinical doctorate (DNP) and focus on being an advanced practice nurse or a clinical leader. Once that decision is made, you need to locate a program that meets your needs and ambitions.

Each school of nursing has selected attributes and strengths that should be investigated and reviewed to ensure you have found a solid match for your educational needs (Clarke, 2016). Some schools of nursing continue to meet on campus, whereas others have moved to the online setting. You may have a strong belief that one method of learning is better than the other. Going to class in a classroom is a traditional mode and may feel more comfortable, whereas online learning provides flexibility around work, home life, and social obligations.

You need to determine whether you will attend school full time or part time and whether your chosen school offers your desired plan (Ketefian & Redman, 2015). A full-time plan of study means you will spend the majority of your time studying, up to 45 or more hours per week. Work and other responsibilities will occur in your spare time. Students who attend full time frequently are recipients of scholarship money through fellowships. Attending part time enables you to work full time to support yourself, although it does lengthen out the time toward graduation.

Other items to consider are cost and the quality of the program. Costs of a doctoral program may include tuition, additional fees and expenses, books, supplies, and money for research and scholarship. Fees at a public collegiate institution tend to be less than at a private collegiate institution, although you should investigate the potential scholarship and fellowship possibilities at both types of institutions. The DNP programs must be accredited by a national accrediting body to demonstrate that national standards have been met. You should ensure that the DNP program is accredited so that you are able to take your required national certification exam to practice as an advanced practice nurse.

Although PhD programs are not nationally certified, you should carefully choose a program that demonstrates indicators of success and has a faculty member who can mentor you in your research topic. Quality indicators of success in PhD programs include the amount of national grant dollars awarded to faculty, faculty productivity in dissemination of knowledge through publication, and the time to students earning their degree (Kim, Park, Park, Khan, & Ketefian, 2014). Your faculty mentor should have expertise in your desired research topic. You will spend significant time with your mentor acquiring knowledge about the research subject and through implementation of your research dissertation so you, as well, will become an expert in the selected field.

CERTIFICATION

Certification is a formal process in which a nurse demonstrates meeting the identified standards of a specific nursing organization in a selected topic area. There are two major paths of certification. The first path is the certification exam that a master's-prepared nurse would take on successful completion of an advanced practice nursing program. This certification would lead a nurse to then practice as a nurse practitioner, clinical nurse specialist, certified nurse midwife, or a certified registered nurse anesthetist (American Nurses Credentialing Center, 2018).

The second path is a specialty certification that may be taken by a registered nurse to validate competency in a selected topic such as critical care, emergency care, cardiac vascular nursing, nurse executive, and more. Kendall-Gallagher, Aiken, Sloane, and Cimiotti (2011) found that hospitals with an increased number of specialty certified nurses had better patient outcomes with decreased morbidity and mortality. Striving for registered nurse specialty certification is now highly encouraged in many hospitals to assist in improving overall health of patients.

CONTINUING EDUCATION

CEUs or credits may typically be earned through attendance at conferences, seminars, or workshops, or with the completion of an article followed by a short quiz either in a journal or from a nursing organization. Typically, every 50 to 60 minutes you spend learning at a conference will result in 1 CEU earned. There are a multitude of nursing organizations that offer a wide variety of topics at conferences at the local, regional, and national levels. You can choose the conference you would like to attend on the basis of the content, location, and cost.

Some states require mandatory CEUs for nursing license renewal. Certifying bodies usually require CEUs as part of the recertification process. The state board or certifying body may have specifications in what topics of CEUs may be necessary; for example, a certifying body may mandate that a certain percentage of the required hours be in the area of pharmacology. In these cases, you will need to maintain documentation of your CEUs earned to demonstrate that you have met this mandatory step.

SELF-DIRECTED LEARNING

Lifelong learning may also be completed through self-directed learning. Self-directed learning activities are those that you choose to complete on the basis of your identified needs through an informal path (Garrison, 1997). You choose the knowledge you would like to informally acquire and then next you choose how you would like to learn that content (Gopee, 2002). The learning activities may be through reading journals, reading professional websites, listening to professional podcasts, or attending in-services or meetings on the basis of topics that you find interesting or may pertain to your job. Self-directed learning may be implemented frequently as you have new questions that arise.

SUMMARY

Lifelong learning is an essential part of every level of nursing. It is important that we stay informed of the latest updates in our discipline to provide the safest and highest quality of care for our patients. Lifelong learning can be accomplished through formal and informal pathways, depending on the type of knowledge and skills needed. As a master's-prepared nurse, it will be necessary for you to continue your learning through many avenues for years to come.

CRITICAL THINKING QUESTIONS

1. What terminal degree option is most appealing to you?

2. Search online for the degree option you would be most interested in. Discuss your findings.

3. What are your plans to maintain a current knowledge base once you have completed your master's degree?

4. What are some strategies you could use to assure the continuing education activities you participate in are of good quality and credible?

REFERENCES

American Nurses Credentialing Center. (2018). ANCC certification center. Retrieved from https://www.nursingworld.org/our-certifications/

Clarke, S. P. (2016). Navigating a research-focused doctoral program in nursing. *Nursing Management, 47*, 19–21. doi:10.1097/01.NUMA.0000475634.98128.83

Collins, J. (2009). Education techniques for lifelong learning: Lifelong learning in the 21st century and beyond. *RadioGraphics, 29*, 613–622. doi:10.1148/rg.292085179

Davis, L., Taylor, H., & Reyes, H. (2014). Lifelong learning in nursing: A Delphi study. *Nurse Education Today, 34*, 441–445. doi:10.1016/j.nedt.2013.04.014

Garrison, D. R. (1997). Self-directed learning: Toward a comprehensive model. *Adult Education Quarterly, 48*, 18–33. doi:10.1177/074171369704800103

Gopee, N. (2002). Human and social capital as facilitators of lifelong learning in nursing. *Nurse Education Today*, *22*, 608–616. doi:10.1016/S0260-6917(02)00139-9

Hicks, R. W., & Patterson, R. (2017). Navigating nursing education. *AORN Journal*, *106*, 523–533. doi:10.1016/j.aorn.2017.10.001

Kendall-Gallagher, D., Aiken, L. H., Sloane, D. M., & Cimiotti, J. P. (2011). Nurse specialty certification, inpatient mortality, and failure to rescue. *Journal of Nursing Scholarship*, *43*, 188–194. doi:10.1111/j.1547-5069.2011.01391.x

Ketefian, S., & Redman, R. W. (2015). A critical examination of developments in nursing doctoral education in the United States. *Revista Latino-Americana de Enfermagem*, *23*, 363–371. doi:10.1590/0104-1169.0797.2566

Kim, M. J., Park, C. G., Park, S. H., Khan, S., & Ketefian, S. (2014). Quality of nursing doctoral education and scholarly performance in U.S. schools of nursing: Strategic areas for improvement. *Journal of Professional Nursing*, *30*, 10–18. doi:10.1016/j.profnurs.2013.06.005

Koper, R., & Tattersall, C. (2004). New directions for lifelong learning using network technologies. *British Journal of Educational Technology*, *35*, 689–700. doi:10.1111/j.1467-8535.2004.00427.x

15

Self-Care

Brenda Scott

OBJECTIVES

1. Recognize the need for self-care.
2. Define maladaptive and adaptive coping mechanisms.
3. Examine various types of maladaptive and adaptive coping mechanisms.
4. Develop a plan to conduct self-care regularly.

Self-care is an important concept in any field of nursing. A good friend of mine regularly reminds me of a perfect scenario that demonstrates the importance of self-care. If you have ever taken a commercial flight, you have heard the safety announcements that include instruction to put an oxygen mask on yourself before helping those around you. Why do you think this is? Is the flight attendant telling you that your life is more important than your fellow passenger? This concept is very important in many more scenarios than just that of an in-flight emergency. You will likely have studied Maslow's hierarchy of needs, and yet we often neglect our own physiological processes to make sure those same needs are met for others. We go for several hours without attending to even our most basic needs such as hydration and elimination. Now, I am not saying to tell a patient, "Sorry I can't help you to the bathroom until after I have my lunch." What I am saying is that you must find ways to prioritize your needs just as you would for anyone in your care. Prioritization is one of the fundamental principles to meet Maslow's hierarchy of needs. We must satisfy those foundational concepts before being able to move up on the pyramid.

Ironically, we teach others how to take care of themselves, yet we struggle sometimes to do those very things ourselves. Unfortunately, just as when patients do not follow our instructions regarding their health, we also face complications when we do not care for ourselves. If you do not take care of yourself, nobody else is going to, and then you will not be able to take care of others. Rose and Glass (2008) described self-care as being able to give yourself permission to take the time to acknowledge and do something about your own health and well-being. Richards (2013) also found that self-care had an impact on positivity and energy, preventing burnout, and improving the patient experience. Richards also acknowledged that self-care is a lifelong journey for nurses (2013). In nursing practice, although we are so focused on caring for others, we must take time and find the right coping skills that meet our own fulfillment and needs.

MALADAPTIVE COPING MECHANISMS

It is not new information that nurses are an unhealthy segment of the workforce. Studies have been conducted for centuries that tell us our own behavior is destructive and leads to maladaptive coping. Maladaptive coping mechanisms are those negative things we do to manage or cope with stressful or traumatic situations. We may drink coffee to provide us energy to deal with a busy day, have a glass of wine to cope with a stressful shift, or withdraw from our family when we have witnessed a traumatic patient situation. These are just a few examples of unhealthy coping mechanisms that lead to negative outcomes. It is important to become aware of these coping mechanisms and address them early. Some are more harmful than others, but each is a means to cover up the true issue at hand. As nurses, it is easy to sweep our needs and concerns under the rug and say we have everything under control. We must develop strategies to address these needs and concerns head-on and quickly.

Substance Abuse

If you have been a nurse for any considerable length of time, you most likely know of at least one nurse who abuses or has abused substances as a method of coping. The most obvious substances that are somewhat socially acceptable and often used as coping mechanisms are caffeine, nicotine, and alcohol. Although many nurses often use these substances routinely, they are not alone. Just a few minutes on social media and you will find some reference to needing a morning cup of coffee before someone can have a civil conversation, or needing a "smoke break," or debating how much wine they may need to consume with dinner to overcome their day. We tend to make jokes and accept these substances, but when we really consider their purpose, they may be covering up critical indicators of coping. At this point in your nursing education, you know the health risks associated with the use of nicotine and alcohol. Caffeine can also pose some potential health risks when consumed in large quantities over long periods of time or combined with health conditions. Even though we are knowledgeable about the side effects, we should pause and consider why we "need" to use these substances. What are we trying to avoid?

Although many may not feel comfortable talking about it, in addition to the above-mentioned socially acceptable substances, there are several legal and illegal substances that are abused by nurses. One thing to realize about substance abuse is that it can happen to anyone. Although some may wish to ignore it or hide it, to see its impact all one needs to do is pick up any state nursing magazine that lists license suspensions and revocations. In any given month, there are likely multiple nurses in your state who have placed their license on the line by indulging in substance abuse. Sadly, this is a growing societal epidemic and many nursing students are even placing their future on the line by abusing substances both on and off the clock.

Currently many employers have a zero-tolerance policy, and because of this many nurses refuse to seek or ask for help for fear of retribution. Because of the prevalence of substance abuse in healthcare, many workplaces and nursing license bodies are realizing that nondisciplinary approaches, treating the substance abuse as a treatable illness, and extensive monitoring allows nurses to recover and return to practice (National Council of State Boards of Nursing, 2018).

Isolation or Withdrawal

In nursing, we see many situations that others cannot begin to comprehend. At the beginning of the early 2000s, studies began to focus on posttraumatic stress disorder (PTSD). In 2007, a study of almost 400 nurses in multiple facilities was conducted by Mealer, Shelton, Berg, Rothbaum, and Moss. This study showed that approximately one-quarter of intensive care and critical care nurses and almost 15% of general nurses had multiple symptoms of PTSD (2007). We all have that one patient or situation that we will remember forever. Can you think of such a situation? Do you remember returning to work after you had the experience? Likely, many of your colleagues continued to discuss the occurrences of the day.

It may become easier to withdraw and place yourself in isolation. Maybe you find yourself spending more time in your patients' rooms or in the medication room, instead of interacting with your coworkers? This behavior would be a warning sign to consider. Withdrawing and isolation do not always show up in the workplace. As nurses, we can withdraw from our family and friends. Have you ever gotten off work, pulled in the driveway at home, and just sat there hoping no one would need you for a while?

A Colleague's Story

Let's look at a story from one of our nursing colleagues. To maintain privacy her name and any personal details have been changed.

After about 10 years in nursing practice, Jane had worked through several phases of burnout. She recalls events that led up to knowing something had to change. She had been working for several years in home health and hospice. There was a period where the company she worked for had, what seemed to her, an overabundance of cancer patients ranging in ages from thirties to fifties. Jane started coming across several scenarios where children about the same age as her children were having to see their parents die. She could see the pain and fear in their eyes. Every day seemed to make her more and more fearful of her own children losing her. She also found herself becoming more and more emotionally unavailable to her own children. Jane often thought the problems her children would share were extremely trivial. Moreover, she started realizing how incredibly unhelpful she was in response to them. She had built some very tall, proverbial, emotional walls to try to protect herself and was hurting those she loved in the process.

This wall became painfully clear one afternoon as Jane was arriving home from an emotionally difficult day. She received a call from another family member. This family member was also having an emotionally difficult day and wanted someone to listen. Her emotional tank was completely empty. Jane responded with "You will have to call your therapist, I do not have time for this today." The minute she hung up, her heart sank. She knew how awful it was for her to say that. Jane knew she just made her loved one feel like a burden and conveyed that she did not really care when she truly did. It was at that moment that Jane knew she needed to stop practicing as a hospice nurse. She could have stayed in practice following some very intentional and in-depth work on her ability to care for herself emotionally. At that time in her life, she did not wish to take the necessary steps toward healing. Instead, she changed specialties.

Nurses face challenges on many levels every day. How we choose to respond helps determine the outcome. In Jane's scenario, she chose to leave a nursing specialty. Social isolation and emotional isolation is not a healthy or helpful response. The process to personal healing can only be defined by you. Although many of us may naturally have this default coping mechanism, you can see how it not only further hurts us but often hurts those around us as well.

Binge Eating

Have you ever had the need to eat some ice cream following that difficult shift? You may have planned to eat only one scoop, but ended up eating the whole carton. How about a couple of slices of pizza and then the whole thing is gone? Binge eating is one common coping mechanism seen in nurses and the population in general. Have you ever heard the term "stress eating"? Stress eating might be described as eating everything in sight when you are nervous or stressing over something. This is a form of binge eating. You may also have heard of emotional eating. This, too, is a form of binge eating. According to the National Eating Disorders Association (2016), binge eating is now the most common eating disorder, and, as of the 2013 *Diagnostic and Statistical Manual of Mental Disorders* (*DSM-5*), has been formally recognized as a disorder. It is important to establish healthy eating habits to avoid binge eating. Developing a healthy and consistent diet is a form of self-care.

Self-Harm

According to the National Alliance on Mental Illness (NAMI), self-harm can include burning, cutting, picking at wounds, pulling hair out, and even breaking bones (NAMI, 2018). Many times, self-harm is easily hidden. You can wear long sleeves to cover cutting, burning, and wounds. It is important to understand that the desire to harm yourself is abnormal. This type of coping mechanism usually requires treatment of some type to overcome.

Sadly, some will not seek help and it will be too late. In our profession, we do not often talk about the ones lost or whom we could not save. We especially do not talk about the ones we lose internally. Although the U.S. statistics on suicide in nursing are woefully out of date, our friends in the United Kingdom recently published statistics showing that from 2011 to 2015 suicide had become the number one leading cause of death below the age of 50 (Office for National Statistics [ONS], 2017). The ONS also found that the risk of suicide among health professionals was 24% higher than the female national average (2017). If that is not scary enough, the ONS noted the reason for this risk was largely because of the high suicide risk among female nurses (2017). If you are dealing with self-harm or thoughts of harming yourself, *please* do not suffer in silence. Let a trusted coworker or friend know. If you are suicidal and need emergency help, call 911 immediately or the National Suicide Prevention Lifeline 24/7 at 1-800-273-8255 in the United States. If you are in another country, you can find a 24/7 hotline (www.iasp.info/resources/Crises_Centres).

Aggression

In the personal story included in the section "A Colleague's Story," you can also see a moment of aggression. Jane was aggressive when telling her family member to contact his or her therapist. Aggression can take on many forms as a maladaptive coping mechanism. This behavior can range from tone of voice to physical aggression. Aggression not only hurts you but also commonly impacts those around you. Many times the aggressive behavior is directly focused on someone you love or even a patient. Again, this behavior is a red flag. If you experience aggression, it is important to identify the cause.

Suppression

Suppression is the most common maladaptive coping mechanism I have found myself using specifically related to nursing. Suppression is burying the painful or traumatic experience like nothing happened, merely moving on from a situation without feeling it. For example, you are working in the emergency department (ED) and a baby is brought in unresponsive. The baby passes away despite several attempts to resuscitate. This outcome is a very traumatic experience. You walk away and avoid talking about the experience. You go to your next patient and begin providing care. You take no time to reflect on the experience. You move on like nothing happened. This example demonstrates suppression. This behavior is unhealthy and can lead to major consequences. You may see burnout as a direct result of continuous suppression.

Compassion fatigue can also be seen in suppression and is another common cause of burnout. During compassion fatigue, caregivers often demonstrate one of two behaviors. The first behavior is obsessiveness, where the nurse becomes obsessive over the care being given to a patient and experiences emotions as a personal trauma. The second behavior is apathy, where the nurse becomes detached, cold, and clinical, and forgets the patient is human and suffering.

Two major defining characteristics within compassion fatigue are time of onset and time of recovery. Compassion fatigue occurs rapidly and, if identified early, can have a faster recovery (American Institute of Stress, 2017). When compassion fatigue is not addressed, it can become another maladaptive coping mechanism manifested in experiences impacting oneself or others. In a longitudinal study founded by the Robert Wood Johnson Foundation and conducted by the RN Work Project, Kovner, Brewer, Fatehi, and Jun (2014) found that almost 18% of newly licensed nurses leave their job in the first year, while approximately one in three leave within 2 years, often because of burnout and compassion fatigue.

ADAPTIVE COPING MECHANISMS

Adaptive coping mechanisms are those strategies that allow you to confront that stressful or traumatic experience with a positive outcome. It is important to identify coping mechanisms before the first experience occurs. You may need a variety of strategies for the different situations you may find yourself in as a nurse.

Exercise

Exercise can be considered an adaptive coping mechanism. You may go walk a few miles to clear your mind after a traumatic experience, take a quick walk around your facility, visit the facility fitness center, play basketball, do Zumba or CrossFit, and so forth. Participating in an organized group exercise program provides not only the benefits of physical activity but also social interaction with those in and outside of nursing. Exercise also stimulates the production of endorphins. Endorphins are the neurotransmitters that make you feel good about situations. If you have ever started a workout routine after being off for a while, you may know this feeling of euphoria. By focusing on the activity at hand, you will likely no longer focus on that traumatic or stressful experience. As with any coping mechanism, if done in extremes it can turn into a maladaptive mechanism. Balance is key!

Meditation

Although there are many misconceptions regarding meditation, there are many types and many effects. Meditation includes multiple forms, including prayer, mindfulness, tai chi, yoga, and many more. According to the National Center for Complementary and Integrative Health (2016), meditation is "mind and body practice that has a long history of use for increasing the calmness and physical relaxation, improving psychological balance, coping with illness, and enhancing overall health and well-being." It is a great coping mechanism because you can do it anywhere at any time. It can also be used as a treatment for a variety of medical conditions.

Commonly, you will want to be in a quiet place. Start by closing your eyes and taking several deep breaths. There are many ways to meditate. There are even applications for the smartphone that will guide you in meditation. I have my meditation app set to remind me several times through the day to stop what I am doing and have a moment to disconnect, breathe, and pray. For me, this moment of silence and breathing greatly increases my productivity. You should try it! Dobkin, Bernardi, and Bagnis (2016) found that healthcare providers who participated in meditation through mindfulness-based stress reduction (MBSR) also experienced more empathy and better judgment in providing patient care. If you won't do it for yourself, would you try it knowing it improves patient care?

Humor

One of the internal mechanisms we have been provided with to help us cope is humor. Humor is probably my most favorite coping mechanism. It seems to be hard to be stressed or traumatized and laughing at the same time. Although we have all likely used humor to get us through some tough situations, the actual scientific evidence showing humor as a coping mechanism is inconclusive. Multiple studies have found that the use of light-hearted humor served as an effective form of emotional regulation, especially when compared with mean-spirited or negative humor (Cann, Zapata, & Davis, 2009; Crawford & Caltabiano, 2011; Kuiper & McHale, 2009; Samson & Gross, 2012). It is amazing what a little laughter can do to stress. Try it!

Journaling

Journaling is a method used by many as an adaptive coping mechanism. This process allows for you to write about your thoughts and feelings. Many times, the journal remains private. Privacy presents an opportunity to be honest about feeling and fears. The key to journaling is the reflection process. Reflection and journaling are discussed in depth in Chapter 13.

SUMMARY

No matter what area of nursing in which you work, it is important to focus on self-care. If you do not invest time in caring for yourself, who will? Determine adaptive coping mechanisms that work for you and keep them close in case you need them. It is important to practice these coping mechanisms so you are comfortable using them in times of stress and trauma. Each person is different, so only you can identify what works best for you. As a colleague once reminded me, your loved ones deserve the best of you, not what is left of you after everything else. Giving those you love your best is only possible with adequate self-care. Remember, you only move up Maslow's pyramid as you satisfy the lower level. Self-care is a key to success, and you deserve it!

CRITICAL THINKING QUESTIONS

1. After reviewing this chapter, what is one new strategy you plan to try as a means of self-care?

2. As a leader in healthcare, how can you encourage others to engage in self-care? What are strategies you can use to open the dialogue with colleagues about self-care?

3. Complete self-reflection identifying any maladaptive coping mechanisms you are using. Reflect on why you may be using these coping mechanisms. What positive coping mechanisms can you use in place of these maladaptive mechanisms?

4. List and define two maladaptive and adaptive coping mechanisms not identified in the chapter.

5. Create a weekly schedule where you include three planned self-care moments. Share your plan with a colleague, friend, or family member.

6. How will self-care influence the environment in which you work? What are the positive impacts and potential barriers?

REFERENCES

American Institute of Stress. (2017). Compassion fatigue. Retrieved from https://www.stress.org/military/for-practitionersleaders/compassion-fatigue/

Cann, A., Zapata, C. L., & Davis, H. B. (2009). Positive and negative styles of humor in communication: Evidence for the importance of considering both styles. *Communication Quarterly, 57*(4), 452–468. doi:10.1080/01463370903313398

Crawford, S. A., & Caltabiano, N. J. (2011). Promoting emotional well-being through the use of humour. *Journal of Positive Psychology, 6*(3), 237–252. doi:10.1080/17439760.2011.577087

Dobkin, P. L., Bernardi, N. F., & Bagnis, C. I. (2016). Enhancing clinicians' well-being and patient-centered care through mindfulness. *Journal of Continuing Education in the Health Professions, 36*(1), 11–16. doi:10.1097/CEH.0000000000000021

Kovner, C. T., Brewer, C. S., Fatehi, F., & Jun, J. (2014). What does nurse turnover rate mean and what is the rate? *Policy, Politics & Nursing Practice, 15*(3-4), 64–71. doi:10.1177/1527154414547953

Kuiper, N. A., & McHale, N. (2009). Humor styles as mediators between self-evaluative standards and psychological well-being. *Journal of Psychology, 143*(4), 359–376. doi:10.3200/JRLP.143.4.359-376

Mealer, M. L., Shelton, A., Berg, B., Rothbaum, B., & Moss, M. (2007). Increased prevalence of post-traumatic stress disorder symptoms in critical care nurses. *American Journal of Respiratory and Critical Care Medicine, 175*(7), 693–697. doi:10.1164/rccm.200606-735OC

National Alliance on Mental Illness. (2018). Self-harm. In *Related conditions*. Retrieved from https://www.nami.org/Learn-More/Mental-Health-Conditions/Related-Conditions/Self-harm

National Center for Complementary and Integrative Health. (2016). Meditation: In depth. Retrieved from https://nccih.nih.gov/health/meditation/overview.htm#hed1

National Council of State Boards of Nursing. (2018). Substance use disorder. In *Practice*. Retrieved from https://www.ncsbn.org/substance-use-disorder.htm

National Eating Disorders Association. (2016). Overview and statistics. In *Binge eating disorder*. Retrieved from https://www.nationaleatingdisorders.org/binge-eating-disorder

Office for National Statistics. (2017). Suicide by occupation, England: 2011 to 2015. Retrieved from https://www.ons.gov.uk/peoplepopulationandcommunity/birthsdeathsandmarriages/deaths/articles/suicidebyoccupation/england2011to2015

Richards, K. (2013). Self-care is a lifelong journey. *Nursing Economic$, 31*(4), 198–202.

Rose, J., & Glass, N. (2008). Enhancing emotional well-being through self-care: The experiences of community health nurses in Australia. *Holistic Nursing Practice, 22*(6), 336–347. doi:10.1097/01.hnp.0000339345.26500.62

Samson, A. C., & Gross, J. J. (2012). Humour as emotion regulation: The differential consequences of negative versus positive humour. *Cognition & Emotion, 26*(2), 375–384. doi:10.1080/02699931.2011.585069

CHAPTER 16

Mentoring

Mindy Thompson

OBJECTIVES

1. Discuss the connection between mentoring and retention.
2. Identify differences between formal and informal mentoring.
3. Compare and contrast role differences between mentor and mentee.
4. Explore key activities of formal mentoring.
5. Distinguish the difference between a preceptor and a mentor.

WHAT IS MENTORING?

Throughout life, you have hopefully had people to encourage, support, and guide you. These people usually have good advice and are people you look to when you are frustrated with a situation. They are also people you admire and respect. They may help you find new paths to explore or help you navigate the path you are on. Commonly, this person is someone who will tell you what you need to hear versus what you want to hear. These people are good examples of what would be considered a mentor. There are some wonderful benefits to both having a mentor and being a mentor.

Outcomes of Mentoring

Have you ever worked somewhere that you felt you had no connection with anyone and were all alone? On the contrary, have you ever worked someplace where you felt like everyone got along well and you knew you could count on others for help if you needed it? In the facility where you felt alone, it is likely you did not have a mentor. You may have relied on a mentor outside the organization. Within this well-connected place, you may have had a mentor. There is a fair amount of literature that suggests mentoring is correlated with job satisfaction, efficacy, productivity, success, and retention (Bruner, Dunbar, Higgins, & Martyn, 2016; Shollen, Bland, Center, Finstad, & Taylor, 2014).

Socialization Through Mentoring

Most large hospital systems now have a thorough orientation process that includes work with a preceptor within the area you will work. Literature also suggests that appropriate orientation can assist in positive job satisfaction ratings and retention through socialization to the new role (Hessler & Ritchie, 2006). Orientation to socialization of role through mentorship can greatly contribute to job satisfaction and ultimately retention. Gilbert and Womack (2012) argue that the commitment to invest time over an extended period leads to true mentorship. The magic is in the time. It takes time to build relationships and trust between people, and trust is the core of a mentoring or any meaningful relationship. Without sincere trust, you likely will never consider a person a mentor.

Furthermore, generalized findings in the literature argue that mentoring and relationship building should be the guiding framework to ensure successful enculturation (Baker, 2010; Gazza & Shellenbarger, 2005). Within every organization, there is a culture of its own along with departments inside organizations having their own culture as well. Having someone you can trust such as a mentor to help you navigate the culture is very helpful in becoming a successful member of the team, department, and organization. Organizational culture is determined by power, politics, and influence (Borkowski, 2015). These dynamics can play key roles in your experience as an employee and the relationships you have within the organization will help determine your role in them.

GENERATION GAPS

With the already identified need for mentorship, one potential issue that may impact retention is a generation gap. Winter and Jackson (2014) completed a study in two cities examining the younger worker employment relationship. Results showed an agreement with human resource management literature in "younger" workers having a different value system than older workers. Some of the differing items in the identified value system include, but are not limited to, the following: a desire to achieve an appropriate work–life balance, an expectation for employers to help fulfill intrinsic work outcomes such as challenging and interesting work, a steady offering of positive

TABLE 16.1 Benefits of Positive Mentoring Experiences

MENTOR	MENTEE
Personal satisfaction	Job satisfaction
Strengthens coaching and leadership skills	Ability to network in academic culture
Opportunity for reflection of own performance through coaching a protégé	Improved performance
Contributes to the success of the entire organization	Increased professional contributions
Creates a legacy	Increased likelihood of retention

Source: Adapted from Bruner, D. W., Dunbar, S., Higgins, M., & Martyn, K. (2016). Benchmarking and gap analysis of faculty mentorship priorities and how well they are met. *Nursing Outlook, 64*(4), 321–331. doi:10.1016/j.outlook.2016.02.008; Holister, L.R. (2001). The benefits of being a mentor: Mentoring enhances your professional life as well as your protégé's. *Healthcare Executive.* Retrieved from http://www.ache.org/newclub/CAREER/MentorArticles/Benefits.cfm; Shollen, S. L., Bland, C. J., Center, B. A., Finstad, D. A., & Taylor, A. L. (2014). Relating mentor type and mentoring behaviors to academic medicine faculty satisfaction and productivity at one medical school. *Academic Medicine, 89*(9), 1267–1275. doi:10.1097/ACM.0000000000000381; van der Weijden, I., Belder, R., van Arensbergen, P., & van den Besselarr, P. (2015). How do young tenured professors benefit from a mentor? *Higher Education, 69,* 275–287. doi:10.1007/s10734-014-9774-5

reinforcement, and high expectations for social interactions and collaboration with coworkers. An additional factor that may inhibit job satisfaction for younger faculty wanting to teach is the salary difference between academic and clinical practice. The American Association of Colleges of Nursing (AACN, 2017) cited the American Academy of Nurse Practitioners as reporting the average salary for nurse practitioners across all specialties as being $91,310, while the average salary for a master's-prepared assistant professor as being $73,633. Keep in mind that these averages are national averages and may not be consistent with what you experience in every geographical area.

As mentioned before, mentoring is a reciprocal relationship with long-lasting benefits for both the mentor and the mentee. Table 16.1 outlines benefits for both the mentor and the mentee.

WHO NEEDS A MENTOR AND WHEN

The easy and short answer here is Everyone! However, the mentor you need early in your career is different than the mentor you need midcareer or even late in your career. You may even find a mentor that sees you through many life experiences. Nonetheless, at every point, a mentor is very helpful.

Preceptor Versus Mentor

Obviously, early in your nursing career you need a preceptor to show you the proverbial ropes. Your preceptor may become your mentor, but this does not happen automatically. A preceptor's primary role and responsibility is to guide you on the how-to's of the job and to orient you to policies, procedures, and so forth. The area of orientation where your preceptor may become a mentor is when he or she helps you understand the political climate where you work in a way to help you mesh with those around you. As you develop a deeper relationship with a preceptor and you receive encouragement, guidance, and advice, he or she is acting more as a mentor. Trust builds over time, and trust is required in a mentor. Remember that mentoring is reciprocal, and this deeper level relationship usually has the mentor interested in your feedback as well. You may hear him or her ask you for feedback on how he or she could help you better understand something or ask you in what other areas he or she can help you. In answering these questions that seem focused on you as the learner, it is also helpful to the mentor.

HOW TO FIND OR BE A MENTOR

Finding a mentor can feel like a daunting task when you are feeling the need for one. However, some of the best mentors tend to just show up and they do not usually introduce themselves as a mentor. You might naturally look to someone in a higher organizational position such as manager and director. These positional leaders may very well be good mentors. However, try not to automatically see them in that role. Remember that meaningful mentoring relationships develop over time. Although leaders or supervisors are definitely people you will want to go to for clarification and advice on certain things, they may not always be the best person to go to for everything (Kaiser, 2017). For example, if you are experiencing conflict among staff at your own organizational level, someone also operating at the same level with experience navigating conflict within that particular set of group dynamics may be a better resource. Again, however, this will require a relationship previously built with trust.

Someone Similar or Different

When choosing a mentor, you could choose either someone who is similar to you or someone very different. There is not a right or wrong answer and the strategy boils down to your goals and your preference. In terms of similarity, you may be using criteria such as age, gender, family stage, career path, or even personality test results such as 5 Dynamics and StrengthsQuest. Some companies have all employees take these assessments, so you may or may not have access to potential mentors within your organization's assessment results. Knowing personality test results could be beneficial if you are looking for a mentor with similar characteristics who has been successful in managing these traits. For example, if you are a new nurse with a young family, having a mentor who either also started nursing with a young family or currently has a young family may be helpful in learning how to manage the demands of a new career with the needs of a young family.

On the reverse, you may be interested in seeking out a mentor who is very different from you. This relationship may work better for mid or late career mentees who have entry-level career navigation experience. An example of when this may be advantageous may be in relation to a personality or working-style inventory as mentioned earlier. For instance, if you have a strong personality trait of jumping into tasks and ideas quickly before asking many questions, you may find value in working with a mentor who tends to ask what may seem to be an overabundance of questions. This person may feel like your complete opposite and may frustrate you initially. However, maturity may allow you to channel this frustration into curiosity to understand how all those questions helps that person be more effective than quickly jumping in without asking questions. This would strengthen your performance if you are able to take your strength and develop it in a way to be more successful. You may learn to quickly begin tasks while simultaneously asking questions, whereas before you began working without any questions at all. Again, there is no right or wrong mentor selection in this regard. The overall objective should be considered to make the best decision for you.

Organizational Impacts

Job satisfaction and retention hinges on mentoring skills of leaders to not only show interest in new employees but also assess individual employee's need for professional development and support of a healthy work environment for all involved (Gutierrez, Candela, & Carver, 2012; Kaiser, 2017; McAllister, Oprescu, & Jones, 2014). Not only do mentoring relationships improve the work environment but there is also indication that they improve organizational commitment in academic settings by achieving a sense of accomplishment (57.4%), autonomy in role (50%), support for professional growth (49.3%), and atmosphere of academic freedom (48.6%; Bittner & O'Connor, 2012). In fact, some would argue that the process of not mentoring new nurses, by way of not acculturating them as new staff, is a form of horizontal violence and incivility (Dunham-Taylor, Lynn, Moore,

McDaniel, & Walker, 2008; Peters, 2014). In response, mentoring and building relationships between nurses should be the guiding framework to secure prosperous employees (Fleig-Palmer & Rathert, 2015). Regardless of whether mentoring is correlated with job satisfaction, efficacy, or productivity, they all have a common result of success and retention (Bruner et al., 2016; Eby, Allen, Evans, Ng, & DuBois, 2008; Felmdan, Arean, Marchall, Lovett, & O'Sullivan, 2010; Shollen et al., 2014).

Group Dynamics and Mentoring

We have touched on group dynamics earlier in this chapter very briefly. Group dynamics among those you work with day in and day out play a big role in finding a mentor or even being a mentor to someone else. Incivility is a very common issue in nursing and has been found to be 10% to 15% higher in healthcare settings than in nonhealthcare settings (Hunt & Marini, 2012). It is also important to note that incivility in nursing is a global problem and not one confined to the United States, as determined by studies on the topic done in various countries around the globe. Although the term incivility is used commonly in nursing, some behavior examples that would be considered incivility include rudeness, condescending remarks, impatience, reluctance or refusal to answer questions, disrespect, and undermining (Roberts, 2015). When you are experiencing these types of interactions, a mentor can be a wonderful guide. You could have a mentor inside the organization who is familiar with the group dynamics and helpful through firsthand knowledge of people in the group. You could also have a mentor outside the organization who is unbiased and also may have experience navigating these types of difficult situations. There is not a one-size-fits-all answer for incivility issues.

Kaiser (2017) highlights empowerment as an effective countermeasure. Empowerment, or the lack thereof, has been found to be a key element of nurse-to-nurse incivility (Laschinger, Cummings, Wong, & Grau, 2014). In addition, nurse empowerment is discussed in Chapter 10 as a way to support nurses in feeling able to be an advocate. When you think of those places you have worked where you felt free to verbalize needs for yourself, others, or patients, these most likely were workplaces where you were supported. In short, you were empowered. Grossman (2013) defined empowerment as the process of providing the tools and resources needed for people to achieve their goals. There is an association between empowerment and positive employment outcomes such as increased job satisfaction, retention, interprofessional collaboration, and autonomy (Bateh & Heyliger, 2014; Kennedy, Hardiker, & Staniland, 2015).

FORMAL MENTORING

Most of the discussion in this chapter so far has been focused on naturally occurring, nonformal mentoring. There are times where a formal mentoring relationship is either requested or assigned. As a master's-prepared nurse, you either may be in a position to be making these assignments or may want to request someone to be a formal mentor. There are some key elements found in literature that would help assure a successful outcome.

The Mentee–Mentor Dyad

Literature offers several suggestions to promote successful mentoring experiences. An overarching theme is meaningful mentor–mentee dyad pairing that results in personal connections that solidify over time and become meaningful for both members of the dyad (Cangelosi, Crocker, & Sorrell, 2009; Grassley & Lambe, 2015; McAllister et al., 2014; Sawatzky & Enns, 2009; White, Brannan, & Wilson, 2010). Another important contributor to successful mentoring is to match mentors and mentees on the basis of goals, interests, age range, and so forth (Grassley & Lambe, 2015; Lasater et al., 2014; Nick et al., 2012; University of California, San Francisco, 2012; University of North Carolina at Chapel Hill, n.d.). Career interests and gender matching has shown to be helpful for female mentees. In addition, race/ethnicity, age, and personal chemistry have shown to be important, but they are hard to predict (Feldman, 2017). Furthermore, the need to create different experiences for nurses on different career tracts is also important to consider (Franko, 2016). Now keep in mind, all of these statements are ideal situations and sometimes you have to do the best with the staff or nurses there are available. Consideration should be given to the possibility of having a mentor outside the organization or department if there does not seem to be an immediately viable option (Tables 16.2 and 16.3).

Mentoring Agreement

To begin a formal mentoring relationship, there should be some communication around expectations. Many times there is a lack of communication around expectations. In addition, there are also times when mentors may not be aware of just what their role should be as a mentor and likewise with mentees. One very important role of a mentee that should be pointed out is the need for the mentee to drive the relationship. As a mentee, you should be sharing what you need. However, sometimes you do not know exactly what it is you need. This is where the role of the mentor can take over with some key questions. We review these in upcoming sections.

TABLE 16.2 Mentor Role Expectations

EXPECTED TO	NOT EXPECTED TO
• Get to know the mentee • Be an active listener • Share knowledge • Help identify the mentee's talents, strengths, and assets • Be open to what the mentee can teach or share with the mentor • Serve as a resource • Allocate time and energy for sessions • Follow through on commitments	• Have an instant rapport with their mentee • Tell their mentee what to do • Seek out a mentee • Be an expert in every area • Have a friendship with their mentee • Do the work for the mentee • Manage the mentee as a supervisor would

Source: Adapted from University of North Carolina, Center for Faculty Excellence. (n.d.). Practical suggestions for mentoring a faculty colleague. Retrieved from http://cfe.unc.edu/mentoring/effective-faculty-mentor/practical-suggestions-mentoring-faculty-colleague/

TABLE 16.3 Mentee Roles

EXPECTED TO	NOT EXPECTED TO
• Take initiative and drive the relationship • Identify goals and desirable outcomes • Seek feedback • Be open to what their mentor can teach or share with the mentee • Be straightforward, honest, respectful, and sincere • Allocate time and energy for sessions • Follow through on commitments	• Be an expert • Always know what questions need to be asked • Have an instant rapport with the mentor • Use their mentor for answers to all their questions • Have a friendship with their mentor • Always do things right the first time

Source: Adapted from University of North Carolina, Center for Faculty Excellence. (n.d.). Practical suggestions for mentoring a faculty colleague. Retrieved from http://cfe.unc.edu/mentoring/effective-faculty-mentor/practical-suggestions-mentoring-faculty-colleague/

When the dyad meets to define expectations, they should also include a discussion of when, how, and how often they will meet. Mentoring meetings may be a casual meeting at a local coffee shop or a standing appointment in an office. However, they could be a phone call, Skype call, Zoom meeting, and so forth. Thanks to current technology, the location of the two people is really not a determinant of ability to mentor someone.

Mentoring Meetings

When the dyad meets, there are some guidelines that will keep the meetings focused, productive, and helpful (Feldman, 2017). As we covered thoroughly in the first sections of this chapter, effective mentoring is built on a relationship. This is true of formal mentoring as well. So, at every mentoring meeting, there should be at least a small amount of time spent on what would be considered "small talk." Take a little time to get to know one another. Get to know the other person in terms of his or her likes, his or her dislikes, his or her family, and so forth. This chat could also include casual conversation about work. As a mentee, be sure to take an interest in your mentor's work outside of what he or she is teaching you directly. What projects is he or she working on? What goals is he or she working toward? Likewise, if you are a mentor to someone, be sure to share some information about your goals and development. People respond and connect to vulnerability. Although menotrs share their strengths through mentoring others, it is also important for mentors to let mentees know about their weaknesses too. One hallmark of a mature leader is the ability to recognize his or her own weaknesses and work around them. This recognition not only demonstrates the ability and importance of self-reflection but also empowers the mentee to do the same that leads to even more growth and development.

After a proportionate short period of time is spent getting to know one another and building the relationship, the next item on the unwritten agenda should be "front burner issues" (Feldman, 2017) These issues are those things the mentees are doing they would rather not be doing, as well as what they have been asked to do they do not want to do. Now, you may be thinking this would just open up the discussion to become a complaining session, but this is where some exceptional help can be offered. The mentor should focus on what the problem is in order to explore ways to work through the challenge. Some examples of solvable issues that may originally present as a complaint may be difficult situations the mentee is unsure how to navigate, work–life balance issues, resource difficulties, and so forth.

These identified issues create a good opportunity to discuss what can be refused and what cannot (Feldman, 2017). We discussed empowerment earlier and this is where the mentor can empower the mentee to create healthy boundaries and balance while understanding there are some things that just have to be done. However, there may be some resources or skills that could be found to help those disliked tasks be done in less painful ways, for example, if a mentee is required to complete a report every week that requires accumulation and calculation of numbers. Perhaps the mentee has found a faster and simplified way to complete the same or similar report and can share his or her process with the mentee, making something that was once a dreadful task to just another item on the to-do list. The mentor should also explore methods of saying no to some requests that protect the mentee's relationship with those making requests. There are lots of ways to say "no" and several ways to do so in a team-oriented manner so the mentee is not seen as difficult by just saying no.

The remainder of the meeting should focus on short- and long-term goals, feedback, clarification, and scheduling of the next meeting (Feldman, 2017). Goals are essential for progression. Mentors can plan an integral role in setting specific, measurable, achievable, realistic, and timely (SMART) goals. Sometimes we set lofty goals but do not take the time to write them out in a SMART format. For instance, as an educator, you may have a goal of "I want to get something published." Getting published, of course, is a great goal. However, without some specifics, it is a hollow goal that is easy to avoid. If the goal was stated in operational and SMART format, it might read more like "I will edit my master's thesis within the next 3 months and submit to xyz nursing journal for publishing." See how the second, SMART, goal statement is action oriented and much more likely to happen? These goals should be written down and discussed at mentoring meetings for accountability as well as support.

As a mentor, one of your first steps may be to help the mentee identify an appropriate journal to submit his or her work to while also sharing knowledge and experience you may have in this area. On the contrary, if you do not have any experience with publishing and feel that you do not have a lot of knowledge, this situation is a good opportunity for the mentoring process to be reciprocal through the mentee sharing what he or she is learning about the publishing process. You are also learning about and feeling empowered to do the same thing. See? It's a win-win!

Another very important activity during mentoring meetings is the exchange of feedback. Obviously, a mentor needs to provide feedback to the mentee to support the mentee's growth and development. Mentors should also seek feedback from the mentee about anything the mentee may notice about the mentor. Although a mentor may feel uncomfortable hearing constructive feedback from the mentee, this feedback presents a wonderful opportunity to learn and grow as a mentor. The mentor has the opportunity to demonstrate the ability of receiving and applying feedback as the mentee is being expected to do. After all, mentoring is a reciprocal relationship where both mentor and mentee should be growing professionally.

Next on the proverbial agenda should be a discussion of what is going well. Here is where accomplishments can be celebrated and strengths can be acknowledged. As a mentor, is there anything you can do to help promote the mentee by informing his or her supervisor of accomplishments? What has the mentee accomplished that could be taken to the next step? Celebrating accomplishments is one way to empower mentees by further building their confidence. What is the mentee not doing but wants to start? Does he or she have an interest he or she has not found a way to connect with yet? How can the mentor facilitate that? Even if the mentor does not have a direct connection to the mentee's interest, experience may provide some thought on how to search out and find those connections. Likewise, the mentor should help the mentee build a professional network. Network building can be done in several ways, such as by introducing the mentee to others, inviting the mentee to professional organization activities, or referring the mentee to known contacts who can support the mentee's goals.

From here, the meeting should be summarized with any tasks to be completed clarified and then the next meeting scheduled. Refer back to the SMART goals, either freshly written or being worked on. What smaller goals can be done between meetings to meet the long-term objective? While considering the frequency and intervals of your meetings, there is no right or wrong answer aside from the following: Meetings should be often enough to satisfy needs of the dyad but not so often that time requirements become a burden to either member of the dyad.

SUMMARY

We come across all types of people throughout life as well as our career. We have discussed what mentoring is, the value of mentoring, how to identify a mentor, and some key elements to a successful formal mentoring relationship. Keep your eyes out for relationships that could become strong mentoring relationships where you are either the mentor or the mentee. Just as we should all have mentors, we should also be a mentor to others throughout every stage of our career. Even as a brand-new nurse, we are leaders. You can probably remember starting out as a new graduate. Today, you could either have years of experience at this point in your career or still be in the first or second year. Either way, you are leading people around you from whatever nursing position you work. From nursing assistants to patients, and to families and communities, we lead by setting an example. Be a good one.

CRITICAL THINKING QUESTIONS

1. Think of a mentor you have had in life. What made him or her someone you respect? How can you incorporate what your respect about that mentor into those to whom you are a mentor?

2. Consider different ways you have declined a request to do something. How did you say no without damaging a relationship? What are some team-oriented ways to say no?

3. Have you ever been assigned a mentor you did not experience a connection with? How did you manage the relationship?

4. Discuss what you see as the difference between a preceptor and a mentor. What value should each role play in the professional development of others?

REFERENCES

American Association of Colleges of Nursing. (2017). Nursing faculty shortage. Retrieved from http://www.aacnnursing.org/News-Information/Fact-Sheets/Nursing-Faculty-Shortage

Baker, S. L. (2010). Nurse educator orientation: Professional development that promotes retention. *Journal of Continuing Education in Nursing, 41*, 413–417. doi:10.3928/00220124-20100503-02

Bateh, J., & Heyliger, W. (2014). Academic administrator leadership styles and the impact on faculty job satisfaction. *Journal of Leadership Education, 13*(3), 34–49. doi:1012806/V13/I3/R3

Bittner, N. P., & O'Connor, M. (2012). Focus on retention: Identifying barriers to nurse faculty satisfaction. *Nursing Education Perspectives, 33*, 251–254. doi:10.5480/1536-5026-33.4.251.

Borkowski, N. (2015). *Organizational behavior in health care* (3rd ed.). Burlington, MA: Jones & Bartlett Learning.

Bruner, D. W., Dunbar, S., Higgins, M., & Martyn, K. (2016). Benchmarking and gap analysis of faculty mentorship priorities and how well they are met. *Nursing Outlook, 64*(4), 321–331. doi:10.1016/j.outlook.2016.02.008

Cangelosi, P. R., Crocker, S., & Sorrell, J. M. (2009). Expert to novice: Clinicians learning new roles as clinical nurse educators. *Nursing Education Perspectives, 30*, 367–371.

Dunham-Taylor, J., Lynn, C., Moore, P., McDaniel, S., & Walker, J. (2008). What goes around comes around: improving faculty retention through more effective mentoring. *Journal of Professional Nursing, 24*, 337–346. doi:10.1016/j.profnurs.2007.10.013

Eby, L. T., Allen, T. D., Evans, S. C., Ng, T., & DuBois, D. (2008). Does mentoring matter? A multidisciplinary meta-analysis comparing mentored and non-mentored individuals. *Journal of Vocational Behavior, 72*, 254–267. doi:10.1016/j.jvb.2007.04.005.

Feldman, M. D. (2017). Faculty mentoring toolkit: UCSF faculty mentoring program. Retrieved from http://academicaffairs.ucsf.edu/ccfl/media/UCSF_Faculty_Mentoring_Program_Toolkit.pdf

Feldman, M.D., Arean, P.A., Marshall, S.J., Lovett, M., & O'Sullivan, P. (2010). Does mentoring matter: results from a survey of faculty mentees at a large health sciences university. *Medical Education Online.* doi: 10.3402/meo.v15i0.5063

Fleig-Palmer, M. M., & Rathert, C. (2015). Interpersonal mentoring and its influence on retention of valued health care workers: The moderating role of affective commitment. *Health Care Management Review, 40*(1), 56–64. doi:10.1097/HMR.0000000000000011

Franko, D. L. (2016). From nothing to something: The nuts and bolts of building a mentoring program in a health sciences college. *Mentoring & Tutoring: Partnership in Learning, 24*(2), 109–123. doi:10.1080/13611267.2016.1178962

Gazza, E. A., & Shellenbarger, T. (2005). Successful enculturation: Strategies for retaining newly hired nursing faculty. *Nurse Educator, 30*, 251–254. doi:10.1097/00006223-200511000-00009

Gilbert, C., & Womack, B. (2012). Successful transition from expert nurse to novice educator? Expert educator: It's about you! *Teaching and Learning in Nursing, 7*, 100–102. doi:10.1016/j.teln.2012.01.004

Grassley, J. S., & Lambe, A. (2015). Easing the transition from clinician to nurse educator: An integrative literature review. *Journal of Nursing Education, 54*(7), 361–366. doi:10.3928/01484834-20150617-01

Grossman, S. C. (2013). *Mentoring in nursing: A dynamic and collaborative process* (2nd ed.). New York, NY: Springer Publishing.

Gutierrez, A. P., Candela, L. L., & Carver, L. (2012). The structural relationships between organizational commitment, global job satisfaction, developmental experiences, work values, organizational support, and person–organization fit among nursing faculty. *Journal of Advanced Nursing, 7*, 1601–1614. doi:10.1111/j.1365-2648.2012.05990.x

Hessler, K., & Ritchie, H. (2006). Recruitment and retention of novice faculty. *Journal of Nursing Education, 45*(5), 150–154. Retrieved from https://www.ncbi.nlm.nih.gov/pubmed/1672249

Holister, L.R. (2001). The benefits of being a mentor: Mentoring enhances your professional life as well as your protégé's. *Healthcare Executive.* Retrieved from http://www.ache.org/newclub/CAREER/MentorArticles/Benefits.cfm

Hunt, C., & Marini, Z. A. (2012). Incivility in the practice environment: A perspective from clinical nursing teachers. *Nurse Education in Practice, 12*, 366–370. doi:10.1016/j.nepr.2012.05.001

Kaiser, J. A. (2017). The relationship between leadership style and nurse-to-nurse incivility: Turning the lens inward. *Journal of Nursing Management, 25*, 110–118. doi:10.1111/jonm.12447. Retrieved from http://onlinelibrary.wiley.com/doi/10.1111/jonm.12447/epdf

Kennedy, S., Hardiker, N., & Staniland, K. (2015). Empowerment an essential ingredient in the clinical environment: A review of the literature. *Nurse Education Today, 35*, 487–492. doi:10.1016/j.nedt.2014.11.014

Lasater, K., Young, P. K., Mitchell, C. G., Delahoyde, T. M., Nick, J. M., & Siktberg, L. (2014). Connecting in distance mentoring: Communication practices that work. *Nurse Education Today, 34*, 501–506. doi:10.1016/j.nedt.2013.07.009

Laschinger, H. K., Cummings, G. G., Wong, C. A., & Grau, A. L. (2014). Resonant leadership and workplace empowerment: The value of positive organizational cultures in reducing workplace incivility. *Nursing Economic$, 32*(1), 5–16.

McAllister, M., Oprescu, F., & Jones, C. (2014). N^{2}E: Envisioning a process to support transition from nurse to educator. *Contemporary Nurse, 46*, 242–250. doi:10.5172/conu.2014.46.2.242

Nick, J. M., Delahoyde, T. M., Del Prato, D., Mitchell, C., Ortiz, J., Ottley, C., ... Siktberg, L. (2012). Best practices in academic mentoring: A model for excellence. *Nursing Research and Practice, 2012*, 937906. doi:10.1155/2012/937906

Peters, A. B. (2014). Faculty to faculty incivility: Experiences of novice nurse faculty in academia. *Journal of Professional Nursing, 30*, 213–227. doi:10.1016/j.profnurs.2013.09.007

Roberts, S. J. (2015). Lateral violence in nursing: A review of the past three decades. *Nursing Science Quarterly, 28*(1), 36–41. doi:10.1177/0894318414558614

Sawatzky, J. A., & Enns, C. L. (2009). A mentoring needs assessment: Validating mentorship in nursing education. *Journal of Professional Nursing, 25*, 145–150. doi:10.1016/j.profnurs.2009.01.003

Shollen, S. L., Bland, C. J., Center, B. A., Finstad, D. A., & Taylor, A. L. (2014). Relating mentor type and mentoring behaviors to academic medicine faculty satisfaction and productivity at one medical school. *Academic Medicine, 89*(9), 1267–1275. doi:10.1097/ACM.0000000000000381

University of North Carolina, Center for Faculty Excellence. (n.d.). Practical suggestions for mentoring a faculty colleague. Retrieved from http://cfe.unc.edu/mentoring/effective-faculty-mentor/practical-suggestions-mentoring-faculty-colleague/

Van der Weijden, I., Belder, R., van Arensbergen, P., & van den Besselarr, P. (2015). How do young tenured professors benefit from a mentor? *Higher Education, 69*, 275–287. doi:10.1007/s10734-014-9774-5

White, A., Brannan, J., & Wilson, C. B. (2010). A mentor–protégé program for new faculty; Part I: Stories of protégés. *Journal of Nursing Education, 49*, 601–607. doi:10.3928/01484834-20100630-04

Winter, R. P., & Jackson, B. A. (2014). Expanding the younger worker employment relationship: Insights from values-based organizations. *Human Resource Management, 53*(2), 311–326. doi:10.1002/hrm.21600

Index